Problem Based Learning in Dermatology

This book presents 15 cases as studies in how to reach a diagnosis from a presenting patient. It covers 15 major topics in clinical dermatology as a succinct reference for dermatology clinicians in practice, also offering a concise revision guide for those in training, from medical students and resident physicians preparing for higher examinations to established physicians in their continuing professional development.

Problem Based Learning in Dermatology

Edited by

Rithi John Chandy MD, MS
Rima I. Ghamrawi DO
Veronica Emmerich MD
Courtney E. Heron MD
Steven R. Feldman MD, PhD
William W. Huang MD, MPH

Department of Dermatology
Wake Forest University School of Medicine
Winston-Salem, North Carolina

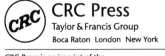

CRC Press
Taylor & Francis Group
Boca Raton London New York

CRC Press is an imprint of the
Taylor & Francis Group, an **informa** business

Designed cover image: Shutterstock

First edition published 2025
by CRC Press
2385 NW Executive Center Drive, Suite 320, Boca Raton FL 33431

and by CRC Press
4 Park Square, Milton Park, Abingdon, Oxon, OX14 4RN

CRC Press is an imprint of Taylor & Francis Group, LLC

© 2025 selection and editorial matter, Rithi J. Chandy, Rima I. Ghamrawi, Veronica Emmerich, Courtney E. Heron, Steven R. Feldman, and William W. Huang; individual chapters, the contributors

ISBN: 978-1-032-57137-9 (hbk)
ISBN: 978-1-032-57136-2 (pbk)
ISBN: 978-1-003-43798-7 (ebk)

DOI: 10.1201/9781003437987

Typeset in Caslon
by Apex CoVantage, LLC

Contents

Preface

In this book, we present 15 patient cases encompassing a spectrum of common conditions in dermatology. Each chapter is distinctively titled with a presenting symptom, inviting you as the reader to examine the clinical image and case description to generate a differential diagnosis before reading the diagnosis. Each clinical case is covered as a succinct reference for dermatology clinicians in practice, while also offering a concise revision guide for those in training, from medical students and resident physicians preparing for higher examinations to established physicians in their continuing professional development.

Acknowledgments

This book was created through the collaborative effort of several physicians and medical students, without whom this book would not have been possible. In addition to the contributing authors, we would like to thank Katie Lovell, Jonathan Greenzaid, and Dr. Christine Ahn for their help with collecting photos for the book. We would also like to thank the publisher, CRC Press/Taylor & Francis Group, for their invaluable assistance in bringing this book to life. Lastly, we would like to thank our patients, who not only entrust us with their care but also enrich our practice with invaluable learning experiences.

About the Editors

Rithi John Chandy, MD, MS, is a PGY-1 resident at AdventHealth Redmond in Rome, Georgia. He earned a bachelor of science degree in neuroscience from Duke University and a master of science degree in biotechnology from Johns Hopkins University. Prior to residency, he completed a dermatology research fellowship under the guidance of Steven R. Feldman, MD, PhD, with the Department of Dermatology at the Wake Forest University School of Medicine.

Veronica Emmerich, MD, is a researcher at the Medical University of South Carolina Department of Dermatology in Charleston, South Carolina. Prior to residency, she completed a dermatology research fellowship under the guidance of Steven R. Feldman, MD, PhD, with the Department of Dermatology at the Wake Forest University School of Medicine.

Steven R. Feldman, MD, PhD, is a professor of dermatology, pathology, and social sciences and health policy and director of the Department of Dermatology at the Wake Forest University School of Medicine. He is the author of several other texts such as *Practical Ways to Improve Patient Adherence*, second edition (2023).

Rima I. Ghamrawi, DO, is a PGY-2 resident at Brookwood Baptist Health in Birmingham, Alabama. Prior to residency, she completed a dermatology research fellowship under the guidance of Steven R. Feldman, MD, PhD, with the Department of Dermatology at the Wake Forest University School of Medicine, during which she authored numerous publications.

Courtney E. Heron, MD, is a PGY-2 resident at Henry Ford Health Department of Dermatology in Detroit, Michigan. Prior to residency, she completed a dermatology research fellowship under the guidance of Steven R. Feldman, MD, PhD, with the Department of Dermatology at the Wake Forest University School of Medicine.

William W. Huang, MD, MPH, was an associate professor of dermatology at the Wake Forest University School of Medicine. He is the editor of other texts such as *Dermatology: Illustrated Clinical Cases* (2016).

Contributors

Jarett Casale
Sampson Regional Medical Center
Campbell University
Clinton, North Carolina

Aditi Chokshi
Nova Southeastern University
Fort Lauderdale, Florida

Isabella Dreyfuss
Nova Southeastern University
Fort Lauderdale, Florida

Megan E. Freeze
Wake Forest University School of
    Medicine
Winston Salem, North Carolina

Roksana Hesari
Lake Erie College of Osteopathic
    Medicine
Erie, Pennsylvania

Saira Khan
Christiana Care
Newark, Delaware

Amanda Krenitsky
University of South Florida
Tampa, Florida

Wendy Li
Harbor-UCLA Medical Center
West Carson, California

Jalal Maghfour
Henry Ford Health System Dermatology
    Department
Detroit, Michigan

Sofia Pedroza
Baylor College of Medicine
Houston, Texas

Varun K. Ranpariya
Wake Forest University School of
    Medicine
Winston Salem, North Carolina

Cristian C. Rivis
Wake Forest University School of
    Medicine
Winston Salem, North Carolina

Jessika Sanz
New York Institute of Technology
   College of Osteopathic Medicine at
   Arkansas State University
Jonesboro, Arkansas

Divya M. Shan
Virginia Commonwealth University
Richmond, Virginia

Brooke W. Sligh
Medical College of
   Georgia
Augusta, Georgia

Josiah Williams
Wake Forest University School of
   Medicine
Winston Salem, North Carolina

1

COMEDONES AND INFLAMMATORY PAPULES ON THE FACE

MEGAN E. FREEZE AND RIMA I. GHAMRAWI

A 15-year-old female presents to the clinic for the first time with erythematous lesions of various stages on the face, chest, and back (Figure 1.1). There are many closed and open comedones as well as numerous inflammatory papules and pustules, but no cystic nodules. The patient's condition started around age 13 and has progressively worsened. It causes her great social anxiety. Previous treatments with benzoyl peroxide–containing facial cleansers and over-the-counter creams were unsuccessful. She has tried reducing "junk foods" in her diet, but reports no improvement. Her condition worsens with stress, such as during important school exams. Family history reveals a mother who displayed similar lesions from age 12 through 26, though the lesions were less severe by age 20.

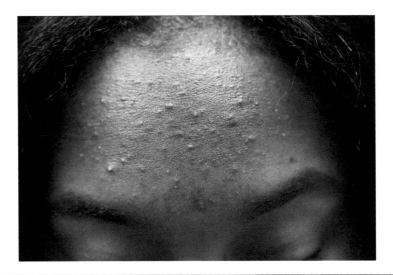

Figure 1.1 Patient presentation.

1. How would you describe the lesions?

There are numerous erythematous, inflammatory papules and pustules as well as erythematous non-inflammatory papules of various sizes.

DOI: 10.1201/9781003437987-1   1

2. What are the differential diagnoses?

There are both non-acneiform (Table 1.1) and acneiform (Table 1.2) conditions that should be considered for this diagnosis. Both types of conditions can be mistaken for acne vulgaris (AV), but acneiform conditions lack comedones. Acneiform conditions are especially important to distinguish from true AV, as they can present similarly. Aspects of the patient's past medical, family, and social history will indicate consideration of these other conditions. These conditions may or may not lack the presence of comedones.[1]

Table 1.1   Non-acneiform Differential Diagnoses

DIAGNOSIS	COMMENTS
Adnexal tumors	Benign follicular tumors presenting as skin-colored facial papules. Though various presentations are found, they distinguish themselves visually from AV by presenting as a single lesion or a small cluster of lesions.[2]
Favre-Racouchot syndrome	Thick yellow skin with multiple cysts and open comedones often seen in older adults. It is associated with exposure to the sun, smoking, and radiation.[3]
Folliculitis	Inflammation of the hair follicle most commonly caused by *Staphylococcus aureus.* These inflammatory lesions may mimic AV in appearance but are often pruritic. AV is differentiated by lesions of various stages as compared to the monomorphous lesions seen in folliculitis.[4]
Nevus comedonicus	Closely grouped, dilated follicular openings plugged by keratinized material that can resemble comedones. This condition is rare and often congenital or develops in childhood.[5]
Perioral dermatitis	Small, clustered erythematous papules in the perioral region with an area of sparing at the vermilion border.[6] AV is differentiated by a more diffuse distribution pattern that is not limited to the perioral area.
Rosacea	Manifests with central erythema, telangiectasias, and papules or pustules on the central face. Typically presents between the ages of 30 and 50 years old and has a recurring eruption and remission pattern.[7,8] AV is differentiated from this diagnosis by the presence of comedones and lack of telangiectasias.[7]
Sebaceous hyperplasia	Umbilicated, yellowish papules on the forehead and cheeks due to visible sebaceous gland enlargement. It is seen commonly in adults with a history of oily skin.[9]
Steatocystoma multiplex	Multiple yellow or skin-colored, sebum-filled cysts on the chest, upper arms, or trunk. It is a rare autosomal dominant or sporadic genetic disorder.[10]

AV: acne vulgaris

Table 1.2   Acneiform Differential Diagnoses

DIAGNOSIS	COMMENTS
Drug-induced acne	Monomorphous inflammatory papules rather than polymorphous papules. Patient will have a history of medication use that is known to cause this reaction[11] (Table 1.3).
Acne cosmetica	Acneiform eruptions appear in association with the application of cosmetics that contain comedogenic ingredients or after excessive facial rubbing such as from sports equipment or an exfoliant cream. Comedones will be present, but the patient will lack a personal history of AV.[1]
EGFR-inhibitor acneiform eruption	Erythematous papules or pustules that appear 2–4 weeks after the patient begins an EGFR inhibitor, such as cetuximab. Lack of comedones distinguishes this from AV.[1]

(Continued)

Table 1.2 (*Continued*)   Acneiform differential diagnoses

DIAGNOSIS	COMMENTS
Occupational acne	Occupational acne can affect all follicles of the body and is associated with an occupational exposure to chemicals such as petroleum and its derivatives and coal tar products or chlorinated compounds. The condition improves upon removal of exposure to the inciting chemical.[12]
Tropical acne	Tropical acne is typically abrupt and arises upon exposure to elevated environmental temperatures. It often manifests as cystic nodules, which can cause scarring.[13]
Radiation acne	Radiotherapy can have various dermatological effects, including acneiform eruptions. Such eruptions can have a comedonal presentation but will be associated with a history of radiation exposure.[14]
Apert syndrome	Congenital disorder characterized by premature fusion of the skull sutures. One of the abnormalities associated with this disorder is inflammatory acneiform eruptions that extend to areas spared by AV. Such areas include the forearms, buttocks, and thighs.[15]

AV: acne vulgaris; **EGFR:** epidermal growth factor receptor

Table 1.3   Common Medications that Cause Drug-Induced AV[11]

Androgens
Azathioprine
Bromides
Corticotropin
Cyclosporine
Disulfiram
EGFR inhibitors
Glucocorticoids
Iodides
Isoniazid
Lithium
Phenytoin
Psoralens
Thiourea
Vitamins B_2, B_6, and B_{12}

EGFR: epidermal growth factor receptor

3. What is the most likely diagnosis?

Given the age of the patient, the most likely diagnosis is AV. AV presents with varying levels of severity but can include open or closed comedones, various non-inflammatory or erythematous inflammatory papules and pustules, and cystic and microcystic nodules. Lesions can present on the face, chest, and back in varying stages, as is seen in this patient. A family history further supports AV, as genetics are believed to contribute to a patient's development and severity of the disorder.

4. What is the next best step?

Careful assessment of the location and types of lesions found on the skin is key to differentiating AV from other acneiform eruptions. Attention to endocrine function is important. Laboratory testing for hyperandrogenism should be conducted in patients with acne and other signs of androgen excess. A thorough history of medications and possible exposures to acne-inducing products is also beneficial to determine the cause and course of treatment.[16]

5. **What are the most appropriate diagnostic modalities (i.e., labs, biopsies, scrapings, histological findings)?**

There are three aspects to diagnosis that may be considered in a patient presenting with potential AV: physical examination, microbiological testing, and endocrinologic testing. During the physical examination, skin should be examined for the type and location of lesions, and any post-inflammatory pigment changes should be noted. This is the most valuable tool in diagnosing and determining the best course of treatment.

Microbiological testing may be considered but is not required because it does not alter the treatment plan. *Propionibacterium acnes*, more recently named *Cutibacterium acnes*, is the primary bacterial culprit in the development of AV. If the acneiform eruptions are non-responsive to treatment or have an unusual distribution, microbiological testing can be useful in distinguishing acneiform eruptions, such as folliculitis, from AV.[16,17]

Endocrinologic testing can also be considered; however, it may also not be necessary, as the role of androgens in the pathogenesis of AV is widely known. Androgen levels will likely be unremarkable unless the patient displays other characteristics of hyperandrogenism, such as early-onset puberty or hirsutism. In that case, further testing may be conducted. These tests include free and total testosterone, androstenedione, dehydroepiandrosterone sulfate (DHEA-S), follicle-stimulating hormone, and luteinizing hormone.[16]

6. **What would you expect to find in the histopathologic analysis?**

Histopathology of AV would show an inflammatory reaction of the pilosebaceous unit. Open comedones and closed comedones are hallmarks of AV and are viewed histologically as dilated follicular cysts containing keratin, cellular debris, and/or inflammatory cells. Open comedones are distinguished from closed comedones by their patent follicular channel to the surface. Other features of this condition include follicular hyperkeratinization, microbial colonization with *C. acnes*, excess sebum production, and both innate and acquired immune responses.[16]

7. **Discuss the epidemiology of this disease.**

   a. **Discuss the incidence and prevalence.**

   The self-reported prevalence of acne in adolescents varies from 35% to over 90%, although post-adolescent AV is relatively common as well.[18,19] Post-adolescent acne prevalence in males and females is 43% and 51%, respectively, for ages 20–29; 20% and 35% for ages 30–39; 12% and 26% for ages 40–49; and 7% and 15% for ages 50 and older. The prevalence of acne in males is higher during adolescence but lower during the post-adolescent years.[18–20] Acne is typically more severe in males, but has an earlier onset in females, a trend thought to be due to earlier onset of puberty in females.[20]

b. **Discuss the sociodemographics of individuals affected by this disease (i.e., age, gender, race, geographic location, other risk factors).**

Although AV is a common condition, various risk factors increase susceptibility to the development of this condition or can exacerbate a patient's severity. External factors such as repetitive scrubbing or picking of the face, chest, or back can rupture comedones and exacerbate inflammatory lesions. Common attire such as turtlenecks, bra straps, and helmets can act in a similar manner and exacerbate or rupture comedones. Styling products that contain pomade, an occlusive agent, may also lead to acneiform lesions.[21]

Some patients believe that diet affects the frequency and severity of their AV. There are several observational studies suggesting that dairy may play a role in aggravating AV. However, no randomized controlled trials have been conducted.[16] Chocolate does not increase the prevalence or severity of acne.[22] However, there are correlations between insulin resistance and AV. Elevated levels of insulin-like growth factor 1 are linked with increased sebum production, which may exacerbate acne.[23]

Genetics and family history are important risk factors and should be determined upon gathering the initial patient history. Having a first-degree relative with a history of moderate-to-severe acne increases a patient's risk by three-fold.[20]

Stress can affect a patient's acne. In one study, although sebum production was not altered during high-stress states, acne severity did increase during times of additional stress, particularly for males.[24]

8. **Discuss the pathogenesis of this disease.**

The pathogenies of AV involves many factors but can be defined by an inflammatory disease affecting the pilosebaceous glands. Lesions begin with abnormal desquamation of keratinocytes at the pilosebaceous unit, creating a microplug, also known as a microcomedo. At the onset of puberty, androgen levels increase and stimulate the production of sebum within the pilosebaceous follicle; these conditions are favorable for the growth of *C. acnes*. This bacteria secretes various inflammatory factors that initiate and perpetuate the erythema and induration and may contribute to hyperproliferation of keratinocytes as well.[25]

9. **What is the clinical presentation of this disease (i.e., grade, stage, subtypes)?**

Clinically, AV begins as a microcomedo that develops into open and closed comedones, inflammatory papules, pustules, and nodules. These lesions are found on areas of the body with the greatest density of pilosebaceous units, namely the face, neck, upper chest, back, and shoulders.[26]

More than 18 classification systems for AV exist that consider factors such as type and severity of acne, number of lesions, location, and quality of life. One of the first classification systems was proposed in 1956. It used four different grades based on clinical observation of comedones, cysts, pustules, inflammatory papules and pustules, and deep lesions that coalesce. Location or spread of the lesions was also considered.[27] More recent classifications grade AV based on photographs and the number of lesions on the face: 0–5 lesions is "mild," 6–20 lesions is "moderate," 21–50 lesions is "severe," and more than 50 lesions is "very severe."[28] However, there is currently no universal classification system for AV. Clinicians may find it most helpful to consistently use one classification system to monitor treatment response. Future acceptance of a universal system will likely maximize reproducibility and ease of use among clinicians.[16]

10. Discuss treatment options.

Treatment of AV is based on four principles: follicular hyperproliferation and abnormal desquamation, increased sebum production, *C. acnes* proliferation, and inflammation.[26] Treatment choice is largely dependent on severity (Tables 1.4 and 1.5) and type of comedone.[16,29]

Table 1.4   Treatment Algorithm for Management of AV in Male Adolescents and Young Adults

	TREATMENT				
AV SEVERITY	BENZOYL PEROXIDE	TOPICAL RETINOID	TOPICAL ANTIBIOTIC	ORAL ANTIBIOTIC	ORAL ISOTRETINOIN
Mild	First line	First line	First line	–	–
Moderate	First line	First line	First line	First line	Alternative
Severe	First line	First line	First line	First line	First line

Note: First-line treatments can be prescribed independently or in combination with other first-line agents. Alternative treatments are often used after failure to achieve adequate response with first-line therapies. These can also be used in combination or independently.

Table 1.5   Treatment Algorithm for Management of AV in Female Adolescents and Young Adults

	TREATMENT					
AV SEVERITY	BENZOYL PEROXIDE	TOPICAL RETINOID	TOPICAL ANTIBIOTIC	ORAL ANTIBIOTIC	ORAL ISOTRETINOIN*	ORAL CONTRACEPTIVE	ORAL SPIRONOLACTONE
Mild	First line	First line	First line	–	–	–	–
Moderate	First line	First line	First line	First line	–	Alternative	Alternative
Severe	First line	First line	First line	First line	Refractory disease	Alternative	Alternative

Note: First-line treatments can be prescribed independently or in combination with other first-line agents. Alternative treatments are often used after failure to achieve adequate response with first-line therapies. These can also be used in combination or independently.

*Isotretinoin is a teratogenic agent. Many physicians will not prescribe this in women of child-bearing age unless severe, refractory disease is present. If disease is severe and refractory to other treatment, women are counseled on the risks of an isotretinoin-exposed pregnancy and are required to either abstain from sex or use two contraceptive methods.

As with the treatment options based on severity, there is a systematic approach to treatment based on comedone type. Treatment for comedonal (non-inflammatory) AV usually begins with a topical retinoid or salicylic acid. If additional treatment is needed, as in the case of mild or mixed AV, a topical antimicrobial (i.e., benzoyl peroxide) or topical antibiotic (i.e., clindamycin or erythromycin) may be added. In moderate papulopustular and mixed AV, an oral antibiotic may be added. An oral contraceptive in females, spironolactone, or oral isotretinoin could be considered next. Severe AV begins with more aggressive treatments or a combination of therapies. Treatments are typically prescribed in a progressive manner until an effective treatment is reached.[16,29]

Since this is the first time this patient is being treated for her moderately severe acne, topical combination therapy is the first-line treatment. It would be appropriate to prescribe topical benzol peroxide and erythromycin in addition to counseling the patient on the importance of daily adherence to the treatment. A scheduled follow-up visit is recommended to monitor the success of the treatment.

11. **Other important questions/details:**
What outcomes can the patient expect and along what timeline?
Patients should expect a realistic timeline to see improvement in their acne. While dependent upon the types of lesions and the course of treatment, improvement is generally seen within 2–3 months. With strict adherence, patients often see results sooner. Adherence can easily be overlooked by both the patient and provider when assessing treatment failure. Various studies suggest that frequent follow-ups can improve adherence rates.[30,31] Adherence rates increase around the time of office visits, making these visits a useful tool to encourage patients to follow treatment plans as well as to avoid unnecessary treatment escalation.[31]

In one randomized controlled study, researchers found that an explicative leaflet plus verbal instructions by the provider (group 2) compared to only verbal instructions by the provider (group 3) was more effective in improving patient adherence and outcomes.[32] The addition of daily reminder text messages (group 1) also proved to be an effective means of treatment adherence and improved patient outcomes. Groups 1 and 2 experienced greater adherences (for 75 and 79 days, respectively), while group 3 was less adherent for 66 days. Group 2 in particular exhibited greater improvement in quality of life as measured by the Cardiff Acne Disability Index (CADI) and the Patient-Doctor Depth-of-Relationship Scale (PDDR) compared to the control group, which received standard instructions, with a change in CADI score of −3 (range −6 to −1) compared to a change of −1 (range −3 to 0).[32]

Patients should be reassured that there are other options if their first treatment combination is truly ineffective or if they experience any dermatological or systemic adverse effects of the treatment. Long-term treatment can conclude with a maintenance prescription of benzol peroxide for occasional lesions and instructions to return if the condition recurs.

References

1. Dessinioti C, Antoniou C, Katsambas A. Acneiform eruptions. *Clin Dermatol.* 2014;32(1):24–34.
2. Zaballos P, Gomez-Martin I, Martin JM, Banuls J. Dermoscopy of adnexal tumors. *Dermatol Clin.* 2018;36(4):397–412.
3. Zheng LQ, Han XC, Huang Y, Li HW, Niu XD. Favre-Racouchot syndrome concurrent with chronic granulomatous reaction. *J Dermatol.* 2014;41(7):642–644.
4. Laureano AC, Schwartz RA, Cohen PJ. Facial bacterial infections: Folliculitis. *Clin Dermatol.* 2014;32(6):711–714.
5. Tchernev G, Ananiev J, Semkova K, Dourmishev LA, Schönlebe J, Wollina U. Nevus comedonicus: An updated review. *Dermatol Ther (Heidelb).* 2013;3(1):33–40.
6. Hafeez ZH. Perioral dermatitis: An update. *Int J Dermatol.* 2003;42(7):514–517.
7. van Zuuren EJ. Rosacea. *N Engl J Med.* 2017;377(18):1754–1764.
8. Elewski BE, Draelos Z, Dreno B, Jansen T, Layton A, Picardo M. Rosacea—global diversity and optimized outcome: proposed international consensus from the Rosacea International Expert Group. *J Eur Acad Dermatol Venereol.* 2011;25(2):188–200.
9. Iacobelli J, Harvey NT, Wood BA. Sebaceous lesions of the skin. *Pathology.* 2017;49(7):688–697.
10. Liu Q, Wu W, Lu J, Wang P, Qiao F. Steatocystoma multiplex is associated with the R94C mutation in the KRT17 gene. *Mol Med Rep.* 2015;12(4):5072–5076.
11. Goldstein S, Wintroub B. *Adverse Cutaneous Reactions to Medication: A Physician's Guide.* New York: CoMedica, Inc.; 1999.
12. Kokelj F. Occupational acne. *Clin Dermatol.* 1992;10(2):213–217.
13. Novy FG, Jr. Tropical acne. *Calif Med.* 1946;65(6):274–277.
14. Turrion Merino L, Vano-Galvan S, Garcia de la Vega MU, Hermosa Zarza E, Garcia del Real CM, Jaen Olasolo P. Localized acneiform eruption following radiotherapy in a patient with breast carcinoma. *Dermatol Online J.* 2014;20(2).
15. Bissacotti Steglich EM, Steglich RB, Melo MM, de Almeida HL, Jr. Extensive acne in Apert syndrome. *Int J Dermatol.* 2016;55(11):e596–e598.
16. Zaenglein AL, Pathy AL, Schlosser BJ, et al. Guidelines of care for the management of acne vulgaris. *J Am Acad Dermatol.* 2016;74(5):945–973.e933.
17. Mourelatos K, Eady EA, Cunliffe WJ, Clark SM, Cove JH. Temporal changes in sebum excretion and propionibacterial colonization in preadolescent children with and without acne. *Br J Dermatol.* 2007;156(1):22–31.
18. Stathakis V, Kilkenny M, Marks R. Descriptive epidemiology of acne vulgaris in the community. *Aust J Dermatol.* 1997;38(3):115–123.
19. Collier CN, Harper JC, Cafardi JA, et al. The prevalence of acne in adults 20 years and older. *J Am Acad Dermatol.* 2008;58(1):56–59.
20. Goulden V, Clark SM, Cunliffe WJ. Post-adolescent acne: A review of clinical features. *Br J Dermatol.* 1997;136(1):66–70.
21. Gollnick H, Cunliffe W, Berson D, et al. Management of acne: A report from a global alliance to improve outcomes in acne. *J Am Acad Dermatol.* 2003;49(1 Suppl):S1–S37.
22. Spencer EH, Ferdowsian HR, Barnard ND. Diet and acne: A review of the evidence. *Int J Dermatol.* 2009;48(4):339–347.
23. Vora S, Ovhal A, Jerajani H, Nair N, Chakrabortty A. Correlation of facial sebum to serum insulin-like growth factor-1 in patients with acne. *Br J Dermatol.* 2008;159(4):990–991.

24. Yosipovitch G, Tang M, Dawn AG, et al. Study of psychological stress, sebum production and acne vulgaris in adolescents. *Acta Derm Venereol.* 2007;87(2):135–139.

25. Webster GF. The pathophysiology of acne. *Cutis.* 2005;76(2 Suppl):4–7.

26. Williams HC, Dellavalle RP, Garner S. Acne vulgaris. *Lancet.* 2012;379(9813):361–372.

27. Witkowski JA, Parish LC. The assessment of acne: An evaluation of grading and lesion counting in the measurement of acne. *Clin Dermatol.* 2004;22(5):394–397.

28. Hayashi N, Akamatsu H, Kawashima M, Acne Study G. Establishment of grading criteria for acne severity. *J Dermatol.* 2008;35(5):255–260.

29. Hauk L. Acne vulgaris: Treatment guidelines from the AAD. *Am Fam Physician.* 2017;95(11):740–741.

30. Feldman SR, Camacho FT, Krejci-Manwaring J, Carroll CL, Balkrishnan R. Adherence to topical therapy increases around the time of office visits. *J Am Acad Dermatol.* 2007;57(1):81–83.

31. Heaton E, Levender MM, Feldman SR. Timing of office visits can be a powerful tool to improve adherence in the treatment of dermatologic conditions. *J Dermatolog Treat.* 2013;24(2):82–88.

32. Donnarumma M, Fattore D, Greco V, et al. How to increase adherence and compliance in acne treatment? A combined strategy of SMS and visual instruction leaflet. *Dermatology.* 2019;235(6):463–470.

2
RED, GRITTY SPOTS

COURTNEY E. HERON AND RIMA I. GHAMRAWI

A 77-year-old white male with a history of hypertension and non-melanoma skin cancer (squamous cell carcinoma treated with Mohs micrographic surgery 3 years prior) presents to the clinic for evaluation of multiple gritty spots on his forehead and cheeks (Figure 2.1). The areas of concern measure between 4 and 8 mm each and are dry, rough, adherent gritty lesions with a slight erythematous background. The patient first noticed the lesions approximately 8 months ago and reports that one lesion in particular has gradually enlarged and feels rougher than when he first noticed it. He reports pruritus and is concerned that the lesions may be skin cancer. The patient has not attempted any treatments.

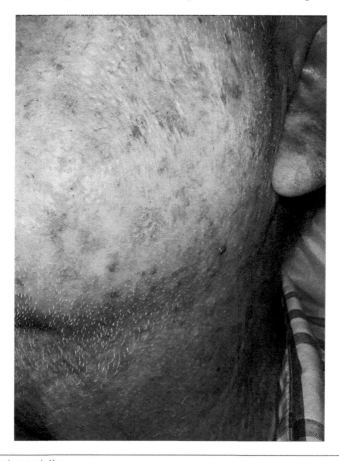

Figure 2.1 Patient presentation.

 DOI: 10.1201/9781003437987-2

1. **How would you describe the lesion?**

   The lesions are 4–8 mm in diameter, slightly erythematous, rough, scaly macules and very thin papules located on the forehead. The biggest lesion is a reddish, 8-mm, thin papule with extensive scale.

2. **What are the differential diagnoses (Table 2.1)?**

Table 2.1   Differential Diagnosis for Red, Gritty Spots

DIAGNOSIS	COMMENTS
Actinic keratosis	AKs are precancerous neoplasms that are due to abnormal keratinocyte proliferation from ultraviolet light exposure. They appear clinically as rough, scaly patches or papules and are commonly found on sun-exposed areas in elderly patients, particularly on the face, scalp, and arms. The margins are often ill-defined, and it may be easier to feel these lesions with a finger than to observe them with the naked eye.[1]
Squamous cell carcinoma	SCCs appear as indurated, scaling nodules or plaques that may ulcerate or bleed. They commonly occur on sun-exposed skin, and over 80% are located on the head and neck. SCCs may also be located on mucous membranes and areas of chronic injury, such as burns or sites of prior radiation. Lesions with deep invasion are often fixated to the underlying tissue.[1] Bowen disease, or SCC in situ, may arise from either a pre-existing AK or de novo.[2] A biopsy is required to definitively distinguish SCC from AK; however, a rapid increase in size, thickness, erythema, ulceration, and pain may suggest progression from AK to SCC.[3]
Seborrheic keratoses	SKs are well-demarcated, oval or round papules that often appear greasy with a "stuck-on" appearance. They may be flesh-colored, tan, brown, or occasionally black in color. Lesions may appear verrucous. The sharply demarcated, "stuck-on" appearance of SKs helps distinguish them from other diagnoses.[1]
Superficial basal cell carcinoma	Superficial BCCs present as erythematous, well-demarcated, oval or round patches most commonly located on the thorax. These lesions may have central erosion or crusting with a rolled, pearly border.[1] The sharp demarcations and often translucent appearance of superficial BCCs help distinguish them from other diagnoses.[2]
Flat wart	Flat warts present as flesh-colored papules 2–5 mm in diameter and may be finely verrucous upon close inspection. Lesions are commonly found in multiples and in a linear formation.[1]

AK: actinic keratosis; **BCC:** basal cell carcinoma; **SCC:** squamous cell carcinoma; **SK:** seborrheic keratoses

3. **What is the most likely diagnosis?**

   The most likely diagnosis in this patient is multiple actinic keratoses (AKs).

4. **What is the next best step?**

   The next best step in the management of these multiple lesions with clinical suspicion for AKs is further evaluation with dermoscopy. Dermoscopy is a useful diagnostic tool for evaluation of AKs; the diagnostic sensitivity and specificity may be as high as 98% and 95%, respectively.[4,5] Any AK that is thick, indurated, or therapeutically unresponsive should be biopsied to rule out squamous cell carcinoma (SCC).[1] Patients should also be counseled on avoidance of sun exposure and other sun-protective measures, including applying sunscreen with sun protection factor (SPF) ≥30 and avoidance of sun exposure during midday (10:00 am to 2:00 pm).[1]

Early diagnosis and treatment are important because of the risk of progression of AKs to invasive SCCs. In select patients with a few superficial lesions, treatment may be delayed, as some AKs undergo spontaneous remission.[6] However, in this patient with a prior history of SCC, treatment should not be delayed.

5. **What are the most appropriate diagnostic modalities (i.e., labs, biopsies, scrapings, histological findings)?**

Dermoscopy may be utilized for enhanced visualization and further lesion analysis.[4] AKs on the body often have surface scaling and dotted vessels, while AKs on the face display a "strawberry pattern," consisting of an erythematous background surrounding the orifices of hair follicles filled with plugs of yellowish, keratotic material.[2] Facial AKs also commonly display white or yellow surface scaling.[4] Furthermore, AKs can be divided into three clinical grades corresponding dermoscopically to three separate patterns (Table 2.2).[4]

Reflectance confocal microscopy (RCM) is another technique that may aid in the diagnosis of AKs, with a resolution similar to histology and a sensitivity and specificity of 80% and 98.6%, respectively.[4] RCM provides horizontal imaging of the epidermis and superficial dermis in a non-invasive manner.[2]

Most AKs are diagnosed based on clinical presentation alone (Table 2.2). Important features of a patient's history include duration of lesion, rate of growth, prior therapies, and family or personal history of skin malignancy. Biopsies should be utilized to rule out SCC when clinical suspicion is high, lesions have been treated previously and are recurrent, or suspicious features are present. The presence of full-thickness keratinocyte atypia is a distinguishing feature between an AK and an SCC in situ.[2]

Table 2.2   Clinical Grades and Dermatoscopic Features of AKs

CLINICAL GRADE OF AKS	DERMATOSCOPIC CHARACTERISTICS[4]	CLINICAL CHARACTERISTICS[6]
Grade 1	• Discrete, white scaling • Erythematous pseudo-network pattern	• Slightly palpable; may be better felt than seen
Grade 2	• Erythematous background with plugs of yellowish material, "strawberry pattern"	• Moderately thick; easily felt and seen
Grade 3	• Profound hyperkeratosis manifesting as a structureless, white-yellow area • Enlarged follicular orifices with keratotic plugs over a scaly, white or yellow background	• Very thick and hyperkeratotic; visibly apparent

6. **What would you expect to find in the histopathologic analysis?**

AKs are confined to the epidermis; thus, lesions may be considered "premalignant" or "precancerous."[2] In SCC in situ, keratinocyte atypia involves the full epidermis, including the stratum granulosum, while the keratinocyte atypia in AKs is typically confined to the lower portion of the epidermis.[2,4] Involvement of the full epidermis in SCC in situ represents a greater disruption of differentiation.[7] The AKs have nuclear pleomorphisms, including enlarged, irregular, and hyperchromic nuclei.[2,7] Additionally, AKs have disorganized growth, which results in disruption of normal differentiation and retained nuclei within a thickened stratum corneum (hyperkeratosis).[7] Parakeratosis, the retention of nuclei in the stratum corneum, is another persistent finding; AKs exhibit focal parakeratosis, while diffuse, confluent parakeratosis is found in SCC in situ. Finally, histopathologic analysis of AKs often reveals alternating patterns of orthokeratosis and parakeratosis, referred to as the "flag" or "pink and blue" sign for alternating eosinophilic columns (parakeratosis) and basophilic columns (orthokeratosis).[2]

7. **Discuss the epidemiology of this disease:**
   a. **Discuss the incidence and prevalence.**
      AKs are quite common in the United States; prevalence is estimated at 12%. It is difficult to ascertain exact incidence, as issues arise regarding diagnostic criteria and diagnostic accuracy in differentiating between an AK and a SCC in situ.[2] Incidence is higher in the southern United States, where there is increased ultraviolet (UV) exposure in general.[1]
   b. **Discuss the sociodemographics of individuals affected by this disease (i.e., age, gender, race, geographic location, other risk factors).**
      AKs may be seen in all races but are most common in individuals with fair skin. AKs are more common in males (3:1 male:female ratio) and individuals greater than 60 years old. High lifetime cumulative sun exposure, immunosuppression, and past history of AKs are other risk factors.[2]

8. **Discuss the pathogenesis of this disease.**
   AKs are the result of intraepithelial damage to keratinocyte DNA, most frequently secondary to UV radiation. In AKs, abnormal replication leads to epidermal cellular hyperplasia with disorganization, increased mitoses, and an abnormal pattern of chromatin.[1] The earliest dysplastic changes in AKs occur within the basal layer of the interfollicular epidermis. Genomic instability in these cells results from inactivation of tumor protein p53 secondary to UVB radiation, which is a pathogenetic mechanism common to both AKs and SCC. Alteration of p53 in these lesions may result in downregulation of Notch 1, a protein expressed in the epidermis that functions as a keratinocyte tumor suppressor and a transcriptional target of p53.[7] Basal cellular atypia may eventually extend upwards to eventually involve the entire epidermis, although some cases remain at the same stage while others spontaneously regress or eventually progress to SCC in situ.[8]

9. **What is the clinical presentation of this disease (i.e., grade, stage, subtypes)?**

Clinical presentation of AKs typically involve 1- to 10-mm, ill-defined, erythematous or reddish-brown macules or thin papules with yellowish-brown, rough, adherent scale.[1] Notably, particularly in early stages, these lesions may be better felt than seen. As lesions advance, they often become better defined and thicker. In individuals with severe photodamage, AKs may form great, confluent patches several centimeters in diameter. AKs are most commonly located on areas of high sun exposure such as the face (malar eminences, nasal bridge, upper forehead, supraorbital ridge), dorsum of the hands and forearms, superior helices of the ears, bald scalp, and shins. Patients may report pain at the lesion site, and importantly, this may indicate that a lesion has evolved into a carcinoma.[2] Three clinical grades are utilized for clinical classification of AKs (Table 2.2). Clinical distinction between early invasive SCC and AKs may be unreliable, and in such cases non-invasive techniques such as palpation and dermoscopy may be helpful to differentiate which lesions should be biopsied.[6]

AKs can be further classified into multiple clinical subtypes beyond the classic variant described (Table 2.3).[2]

Table 2.3 Additional Clinical Subtypes of AKs

CLINICAL SUBTYPE	CHARACTERISTICS
Actinic cheilitis	• Actinic cheilitis refers to characteristic changes that occur on the lower lip as a result of moderate-to-severe photodamage.[2] • Presentation varies from well-defined, erythematous papules and plaques with scale to diffuse erythema and scale with possible areas of leukoplakia.[2] • Potential for transformation to SCC is higher than for other subtypes of AK.[2]
Atrophic	• Erythematous or pink macules or patches with slight scale.[2]
Hypertrophic	• Papules and plaques with an erythematous base and hyperkeratotic scale.[2] • Thickness of lesion is often bothersome to patients.[2] • Cutaneous horns may develop; these should be biopsied for underlying malignancy.[2]
Lichenoid	• Presents similarly to classic AKs but has a greater degree of erythema around the base of the lesion.[2] • Patients may experience tenderness or pruritus in a pre-existing AK at the onset of the dermal inflammatory infiltrate associated with this subtype.[2]
Pigmented	• Lesions may lack erythema and often have a reticulated or hyperpigmented appearance.[2] • Dermoscopy may help distinguish pigmented AKs from lentigines, reticulated seborrheic keratosis, or lentigo maligna melanomas.[2]

AK: actinic keratosis; **AKs:** actinic keratoses; **SCC:** squamous cell carcinoma

10. **Discuss treatment options.**

Treatment may be either lesion-directed or field-directed (Table 2.4). Lesion-directed therapy is indicated for lesions that are few in number and isolated, while field-directed therapy is indicated for multiple lesions located on areas of sun-damaged skin with a high likelihood of subclinical lesions. Field-directed therapy frequently results in considerable discomfort to patients post-treatment as a result of treatment-induced inflammation.[9] In the case of this patient with multiple lesions, field-directed therapy is likely the best choice. Lesion-directed therapy using cryosurgery with liquid nitrogen could be used in addition to field-directed therapy for the larger lesions, as this is the treatment of choice when few lesions are present.[1,2]

Table 2.4   Treatment Options for AKs

TREATMENT TYPE	TREATMENT	INDICATIONS	MECHANISM OF ACTION	NOTES
Lesion-directed therapy	Curettage with electrodessication	Thick, hypertrophic lesions[9]	Removal of diseased tissue with a curette followed by cautery at site	• Lesions often heal with a hypopigmented scar.[2]
	Liquid nitrogen cryosurgery	Isolated or few lesions	Freezing causes separation of the epidermis and dermis	• Attempting to freeze thicker lesions may result in untreated cells at lesion base.[9] • Treatment may result in residual hypopigmentation, especially in lesions of darker-skinned patients.[9]
	Surgical removal (shave excision)	Lesions with thick crust or induration[9]	Removal of diseased tissue with a minor surgical procedure	• Small, thicker lesions may be better removed with curettage and electrodessication. • Lesions often heal with hypopigmented scar.[2] • Lesions <0.5 cm do not require biopsy.[9]
Field-directed therapy	Diclofenac	Multiple AKs in sun-damaged skin	Blocks COX-2, reducing inflammation and cellular proliferation; induces cellular apoptosis[10]	• Treatment period is 90 days.[2] • May result in a less severe cutaneous reaction than other field-directed therapies.[10] • Duration of therapy may result in concerns with adherence.[2]
	Ingenol mebutate	Multiple AKs in sun-damaged skin	Results in rapid cell death of tumor cells[9]	• Extracted from the sap of the *Euphorbia peplus* plant.[9] • Works quickly; healing occurs approximately 10–14 days post-treatment initiation.[2] • Supposedly does not result in residual hypopigmentation.[2]
	Photodynamic therapy	Multiple AKs in sun-damaged skin	Damaged cells undergo a toxic photochemical reaction[9]	• Must avoid sun exposure for 48 hours post-treatment.[2] • Works quickly, with recovery 1–2 weeks post-treatment.[2]

(Continued)

Table 2.4 (*Continued*)   Treatment Options for AKs

TREATMENT TYPE	TREATMENT	INDICATIONS	MECHANISM OF ACTION	NOTES
	Topical chemotherapy with 5-FU	Superficial AKs	5-FU inhibits the enzyme thymidylate synthase, blocking DNA replication[1]	• Results in inflammation, which is greater in thicker, more indurated lesions.[9] • Patients may experience considerable discomfort post-treatment as a result of inflammation. • The most commonly utilized regimen is 5-FU cream 5%, applied twice daily for 2–4 weeks.[1] • May result in potentially severe photosensitivity.[2]
	Topical chemotherapy with imiquimod cream	Multiple AKs in sun-damaged skin	Functions as an immune response modifier[1]	• May result in flu-like symptoms.[2] • Lesions may heal with hypopigmented scar.[2] • Not recommended for patients with an underlying autoimmune condition.[2]

AKs: actinic keratoses; **COX-2:** cyclo-oxygenase-2; **5-FU:** 5-fluorouracil; **Th1:** type 1 T helper cell; **TLR-7:** Toll-like receptor 7

11. **Other important questions/details:**
    Risk of transformation of AK to SCC
    For any given AK, the likelihood of transformation to an invasive SCC is estimated to occur at a rate of 0.075–0.096% per lesion per year.[2] For AKs that do transform to invasive SCC, the average length of time for progression is approximately 2 years.[9]
    Risk factors associated with transformation of AK to SCC
    Risk factors associated with malignant transformation of AKs include lesions located on the lips, ears, trunk, and lower extremities. Additional risk factors include lesion diameter >1 cm and a lesion history of ulceration, bleeding, and erythema.[9]

References

1. Marks J, Miller J. *Lookingbill & Marks' Principles of Dermatology*. 5th ed. Elsevier; 2013.
2. Bolognia J, Schaffer J, Cerroni L. *Dermatology*. 4th ed. Elsevier; 2018.
3. Moy RL. Clinical presentation of actinic keratoses and squamous cell carcinoma. *J Am Acad Dermatol*. 2000;42(1 Pt 2):8–10.
4. Casari A, Chester J, Pellacani G. Actinic keratosis and non-invasive diagnostic techniques: An update. *Biomedicines*. 2018;6(1).
5. Zalaudek I, Giacomel J, Argenziano G, et al. Dermoscopy of facial nonpigmented actinic keratosis. *Br J Dermatol*. 2006;155(5):951–956.

6. Zalaudek I, Piana S, Moscarella E, et al. Morphologic grading and treatment of facial actinic keratosis. *Clin Dermatol.* 2014;32(1):80–87.

7. Ratushny V, Gober MD, Hick R, Ridky TW, Seykora JT. From keratinocyte to cancer: The pathogenesis and modeling of cutaneous squamous cell carcinoma. *J Clin Invest.* 2012;122(2):464–472.

8. Fernandez Figueras MT. From actinic keratosis to squamous cell carcinoma: Pathophysiology revisited. *J Eur Acad Dermatol Venereol.* 2017;31(Suppl 2):5–7.

9. Dinulos J. *Habif's Clinical Dermatology.* Elsevier; 2020.

10. Nelson CG. Diclofenac gel in the treatment of actinic keratoses. *Ther Clin Risk Manag.* 2011;7:207–211.

3

ITCHY, RED RASH ON ELBOWS AND BACK OF KNEES

AMANDA KRENITSKY AND WENDY LI

A 13-year-old female with a history of asthma presents to the clinic with an itchy, red rash on the inside of both elbows and the back of both knees (Figure 3.1). The rash has been intermittent for the past few years and is noticeably worse in the winter. She reports applying over-the-counter hydrocortisone ointment on the affected areas with minimal improvement. She does not use any moisturizers.

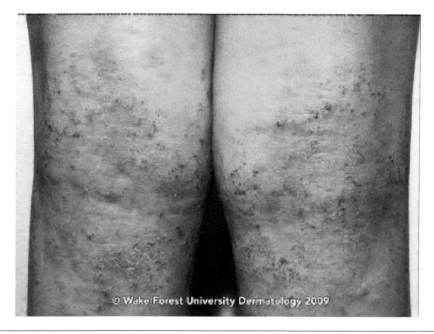

Figure 3.1 Patient presentation.

1. **How would you describe the lesion(s)?**
   Multiple poorly defined, 1- to 1.5-cm, erythematous, thin papules and plaques with lichenification in the bilateral antecubital and popliteal fossae.

DOI: 10.1201/9781003437987-3

2. What are the differential diagnoses (Table 3.1)?

Table 3.1 Differential Diagnoses for Itchy, Red Rash on Elbows and Back of Knees

DIAGNOSIS	COMMENTS
Atopic dermatitis (AD)	Most commonly affects children, but can occur at any age. Clinical features include erythematous papules and plaques with or without scaling and crusting. Areas affected vary based on age: • *Infants/young children:* extensor surfaces, cheeks or scalp, with relative sparing of the diaper area • *Older children and adolescents:* antecubital and popliteal fossae, volar aspect of wrists, ankles, and neck • *Adults:* flexor surfaces, hands, face, or neck Clinical presentation and features of eczematous lesions vary based on stage of disease (acute/subacute/chronic).[1]
Allergic or irritant contact dermatitis	Contact dermatitis presents with erythematous papules and plaques, with or without crust and scale, following exposure to an allergen or irritant and can occur at any age. The lesions are classically focal, patterned, and confined to the site of exposure. Allergic contact dermatitis has a delayed onset, whereas irritant contact dermatitis develops rapidly within a few hours of exposure.[1]
Seborrheic dermatitis	Seborrheic dermatitis presents as poorly demarcated, erythematous patches and thin plaques with greasy scale and is often associated with pruritus. These lesions may present at any age. In infants, the scalp is affected, and is referred to as "cradle cap." In adults, hair-bearing areas of the face, such as eyebrows, ears, or beard areas, are commonly affected in addition to the scalp.[1]
Psoriasis	Psoriasis presents as well-demarcated, erythematous plaques with micaceous, silvery scale. Peak age of onset is bimodal, occurring most commonly between 30–39 years and 50–69 years of age. In infants, disease typically involves the diaper area; in adolescents and adults, the scalp, elbows, and knees are commonly affected.[1]
Scabies	Scabies presents as diffuse, erythematous papules with or without excoriations and crust. Burrows may also be visible. Nearly any area of the body may be affected, with frequent involvement of intertriginous areas as well as palms and soles. The back and head are relatively spared, other than in young children. The presence of vesiculopustular lesions on the palms and soles and involvement of skin folds in infants suggest the diagnosis of scabies.[1]
Mycosis fungoides (MF)	Mycosis fungoides presents as erythematous and scaly patches or plaques, most commonly located on the trunk. Peak age of onset is between 55 and 60 years, though it can occur in patients under 35 years as well.[2]

Less common diagnoses to consider include drug reactions, primary immuno-deficiencies (Wiskott-Aldrich syndrome, hyperimmunoglobulin E syndrome), nutritional deficiencies (zinc, pyridoxine, niacin), Netherton syndrome, and cutaneous T-cell lymphoma.[1]

3. What is the most likely diagnosis?

The most likely diagnosis for this patient is atopic dermatitis (AD), also known as eczema.

4. What is the next best step?

The next best step in the management of this patient is to obtain an adequate personal and family history in an attempt to discern the temporal course and potential triggers as well as any familial history of atopy. A thorough skin exam should be performed, looking for the common characteristic features of AD as well as any associated features, or "atopic stigmata" (xerosis, ichthyosis vulgaris, keratosis pilaris, palmar and plantar hyperlinearity, Dennie-Morgan lines, periorbital darkening, anterior neck folds, white dermographism, follicular prominence).[1] The history and physical exam findings are not only important for the diagnosis of AD but will also help guide the individual treatment plan.

5. **What are the most appropriate diagnostic modalities (i.e., labs, biopsies, scrapings, histological findings)?**

AD is typically a clinical diagnosis, based on history and physical exam findings (morphology and distribution of skin lesions) and associated clinical signs. Skin culture with antibiotic susceptibility may be considered if superinfection is suspected.[3]

Diagnostic criteria for AD encompass one mandatory and five major criteria. A diagnosis of AD is made when a patient experiences pruritus (mandatory criteria) plus three or more of the major criteria. Major criteria include involvement of the skin creases, personal history of asthma or hay fever (or family history of AD in a first-degree relative if the patient is under 4 years of age), dry skin within the last year, presence of symptoms in a child prior to 2 years of age, or visible dermatitis involving the areas relevant to the patient's age group.[4,5]

If the diagnosis is unclear, a skin biopsy, serum immunoglobulin E (IgE) level, potassium hydroxide (KOH) preparation, allergen patch testing, genetic testing, and/or human immunodeficiency virus (HIV) testing may be performed for confirmation and to rule out other skin conditions. These tests, however, are not routinely utilized in the diagnosis of AD.[1,3] It is important to note that in adults with persistent or treatment-resistant AD, a skin biopsy should be performed to rule out mycosis fungoides, a cutaneous T-cell lymphoma with a clinical presentation similar to that of AD.[1,2]

6. **What would you expect to find in the histopathologic analysis?**

Skin biopsy findings will vary based on the stage of AD as well as the location of the biopsy. In subclinical AD, a skin biopsy will reveal sparse perivascular T-cell infiltrates. Characteristic histopathologic findings of acute AD lesions include mild acanthosis, epidermal spongiosis, lymphocytic exocytosis, an abundance of antigen presenting in the superficial dermis, and eosinophilia. Chronic or lichenified lesions have the characteristic findings of an acanthotic epidermis with rete ridge elongation, parakeratosis, minimal spongiosis, abundant IgE-bearing antigen-presenting cells, macrophage-dominant mononuclear cell dermal infiltrate, and marked eosinophilia.[6]

7. **Discuss the epidemiology of this disease.**

   a. **Discuss the incidence and prevalence:**

   Since the 1970s, the incidence of AD has increased by nearly threefold. Approximately 15–20% of children and 1–3% of adults are affected worldwide. Within the United States, the prevalence of AD is approximately 10.7% and 7.2% for children and adults, respectively.[1]

a. **Discuss the sociodemographics of individuals affected by this disease (i.e., age, gender, race, geographic location, other risk factors):**
Although onset of AD can occur at any age, children are most commonly affected. Of those affected, 60% of patients will develop the condition within their first year of life, and 90% of patients will develop it by the age of 5 years. The majority of patients are clear of AD by late childhood; however, the disease may persist into adolescence and adulthood.[1]

8. **Discuss the pathogenesis of this disease.**
The exact cause of AD is not definitively known; however, the development of epidermal barrier dysfunction and cutaneous inflammation are postulated to be secondary to the interplay of various genetic, immunologic, and environmental or lifestyle factors that result in epidermal barrier dysfunction and cutaneous inflammation.[7]

Major genetic risk factors for AD include a family history of atopy and a loss-of-function mutation in the filaggrin gene (FLG) leading to reduced levels of filaggrin, an epidermal structural protein.[8,9] Genetic association studies suggest involvement of the *SPINK5* gene, which codes for a lymphoepithelial Kazal-type protease inhibitor (LEKT1) that is involved in the processing of profilaggrin into filaggrin in the pathogenesis of AD.[10,11] New susceptibility loci for AD have been described, including 5q31 (*KIF3A*), 11q13 (*OVOLI*), and 19p13 (*ADAMS10/ACTL9*).[12–15] These genetic mutations result in loss or dysfunction of filaggrin as well as other stratum corneum proteins—such as corneodesmosin, desmoglein-1, desmocollin-1, transglutaminase-3, and tight junction-related proteins—ultimately leading to skin barrier dysfunction.[1,16]

In AD, the immune system inappropriately responds to skin surface antigens, resulting in cutaneous inflammation. There are a number of proposed mechanisms, involving both the innate and adaptive immune systems, by which this occurs. Patients with AD have reduced toll-like receptor (TLR)-2 and TLR-9 function, leading to a defect in their innate immune-mediated epidermal repair function, alteration in the microbiome of the skin, and additional inflammation, and hence, greater risk of bacterial superinfection.[1,17–19] The adaptive immune response is also involved, as the enhanced allergen penetration through an impaired skin barrier resulting in a type 2 helper (Th2) T lymphocyte–type milieu is a proposed critical link between the primary barrier defect in AD and Th2 polarization.[20,21] Thymic stromal lymphopoietin (TSLP) polymorphisms are potential markers of disease severity.[22,23]

While not a direct cause of AD, environmental and lifestyle factors such as inappropriate bathing habits (i.e., long hot showers), sweating, environmental allergens, heat, humidity, fragrance-containing soaps and detergents, abrasive clothing, chemicals, smoke, and stress may play a role in the triggering and exacerbation of this condition.[1]

9. **What is the clinical presentation of this disease (i.e., grade, stage, subtypes)?**

Presentation of AD can vary by age. Infants and toddlers are commonly affected on the scalp, forehead, cheeks, and extensor surfaces. Adolescents and adults are commonly affected on flexural surfaces of the neck, elbows, wrists, knees, and ankles.[1,24]

There are three stages of AD: acute, subacute, and chronic. Acute lesions of AD present as erythematous papules coalescing into plaques. Secondary changes may include weeping, crusting, or scaling. Subacute lesions of AD present as red, dry, scaly patches or papules with or without crust or scale. Chronic AD follows a relapsing course over months to years. Patients present with poorly demarcated, diffusely dry, and erythematous skin lesions. Characteristic features of chronic AD include lichenification, hyperpigmentation, and scale.[1,24]

Intense pruritus is a hallmark symptom of AD. Scratching of the lesions leads to the secondary epithelial changes seen in chronic AD, as well as increased risk of cutaneous infection. Patients with AD are predisposed to the development of bacterial and viral skin infections. Because *Staphylococcus aureus* colonizes nearly 100% of AD patients, impetiginization of AD lesions frequently occurs and is associated with disease exacerbation. Hemorrhagic crusts can be indicative of superinfection in these patients.[1,25–27]

There is a plethora of methods for rating the severity of disease in patients with AD, including the SCORing Atopic Dermatitis (SCORAD) index; Eczema Area and Severity Index (EASI); Patient-Oriented Eczema Measure (POEM); Six Area, Six Sign Atopic Dermatitis (SASSAD) severity score; and the Investigator's Global Assessment (IGA).[3,28] However, while these severity scores are extremely useful for research purposes, there is minimal indication for their use in clinical practice. Clinically, disease severity is subjectively measured by the clinician based on each patient's symptoms (i.e., pruritus, impact on sleep and daily activities) to assess individual treatment plan needs.

10. **Discuss treatment options.**

First-line treatment of mild-to-moderate AD is topical corticosteroids (Table 3.2). The potency of the steroid prescribed is dependent on the location of the lesions and can be delivered via different vehicles (Table 3.3). For disease localized to the trunk, mid- or high-potency steroids may be used. Low-potency steroids should be used for the treatment of mild-to-moderate AD involving the face, intertriginous areas, or other regions with thinner skin. With good adherence to treatment, topical corticosteroids are a very efficacious treatment for AD. The main adverse effects associated with long-term use of these medications include skin atrophy, pigmentation changes, or the development of striae. Other topical medications—such as topical calcineurin inhibitors (tacrolimus, pimecrolimus) and phosphodiesterase-4 inhibitors (crisaborole)—are useful alternatives to topical corticosteroids for mild-to-moderate AD involving the face, eyes, neck, and intertriginous body areas. The main benefit of these alternative topical treatments is that they offer comparable efficacy in treatment of delicate areas without the adverse effect profile of topical corticosteroids.[1,24]

Table 3.2   Potency Classes of Topical Corticosteroids

POTENCY	CLASS	GENERIC NAME	FORMULATIONS
Very high	I	Betamethasone dipropionate	0.05% G O
		Clobetasol	0.05% C F G L O
		Halobetasol propionate	0.05% C O
High	II	Betamethasone dipropionate	0.05% C
		Desoximetasone	0.05% G
			0.25% C O
		Fluocinonide	0.05% C G O S
		Mometasone furoate	0.10% O
	III	Betamethasone dipropionate	0.05% C
		Betamethasone valerate	0.10% O
		Desoximetasone	0.05% C
		Fluticasone propionate	0.005% O
		Halcinonide	0.10% O S
		Triamcinolone	0.10% O
Mid	IV	Betamethasone valerate	0.12% F
		Fluocinolone acetonide	0.025% O
		Hydrocortisone valerate	0.20% O
		Mometasone furoate	0.10% C
		Triamcinolone	0.10% C
	V	Betamethasone dipropionate	0.05% L
		Betamethasone valerate	0.10% C
		Fluocinolone acetonide	0.025% C
		Hydrocortisone butyrate	0.10% C
		Hydrocortisone valerate	0.20% C
Low	VI	Betamethasone valerate	0.10% L
		Desonide	0.05% C L O
		Fluocinolone acetonide	0.01% C S
	VII	Hydrocortisone acetate	0.50% C L O
			1.00% C F O
		Hydrocortisone hydrochloride	0.25% C L
			0.50% C L O S
			100% C L O S
			2.0% L
			2.5% C L O S

C: cream; **F:** foam; **G:** gel; **L:** lotion; **O:** ointmentss

Table 3.3 Vehicles of Topical Corticosteroids

PREPARATION	COMPOSITION	EFFECT ON SKIN	CHARACTERISTICS
Ointment	Water in oil emulsion	Moisturizing	Most potent and has occlusive property for inducing skin hydration; greasy and limited utility in hairy areas
Cream	Oil in water emulsion	Moisturizing	Most commonly prescribed
Lotion	Oil in water emulsion	Drying	Least potent; effective at cooling and soothing; good patient compliance
Solution	Alcohol	Drying	Scalp use
Gel	Propylene glycol and water	Drying	Easy application, good patient compliance, lack of irritating components

For AD that is moderate to severe, extensive, and/or resistant to treatments with topical steroids, a number of systemic treatments are available. Dupilumab is a fully human monoclonal antibody that binds to the α subunit of the interleukin (IL)-4 receptor and inhibits downstream signaling of IL-4 and IL-13, both cytokines of the Th2 lymphocyte immune response pathway. Clinical trials also support the use of dupilumab in adults with severe AD who are unresponsive to topical therapies alone and in whom other systemic treatments are contraindicated.[29–31] Other available systemic immunosuppressant agents, including cyclosporine, methotrexate, azathioprine, and mycophenolate mofetil, may also be used. Additionally, phototherapy is a highly effective treatment modality for moderate-to-severe AD.[1,24,32–34] Narrowband ultraviolet (UV) B, UVA, psoralen + UVA, and UVA_1 are among the various types of phototherapy, and are often used alone or in combination with various topical and systemic treatments.

Treatment of AD consists of long-term therapy to help control symptoms and decrease frequency of flares. Maintenance of treatment and prevention of exacerbations are crucial aspects of AD treatment, regardless of severity. Proper skin care is achieved with lukewarm baths; use of mild, fragrance-free cleansers, moisturizers, and emollients to protect the skin barrier; and identifying and avoiding irritants. Medication adherence is fundamental to successful treatment outcomes. Poor adherence is a frequent barrier to effective treatment, with particularly poor adherence to topical medications. Factors affecting adherence may include medication cost, pharmacy access, ability to execute treatment initiation and maintenance (e.g., patient age and cognitive ability), and fear of adverse effects. It is important to acknowledge such limiting factors when formulating a treatment plan and to be able to implement practices that can improve adherence, such as frequent follow-up visits.[13,35,36,40] An important aspect of treatment to consider in patients with AD is the associated pruritus. The treatment for pruritus consists of oral antihistamines. However, because these medications are associated with adverse effects such as drowsiness, they are not considered first-line. Antihistamine therapy may be considered for individuals who experience disruption of sleep, as this is common in patients experiencing the intense pruritus at night. The drowsiness induced by antihistamines is beneficial and improves the quality of life of both the patient and their family members. Oral non-sedating antihistamines are useful in patients with concomitant allergic symptoms such as urticaria, dermographism, or allergic conjunctivitis.[1,32]

Patients with AD are predisposed to the development of secondary bacterial and viral infections of the skin. In instances of superimposed bacterial infection, *S. aureus* is the most common causative agent; as such, antibiotic treatment covering this organism is indicated in addition to topical or intranasal mupirocin.[1] Bleach baths diluted in a 1:4 to 1:2 bleach:water ratio may be useful in patients at higher risk of infection, such as those with a history of superinfection or those with multiple excoriations. Superinfection with viruses such as herpes simplex virus (eczema herpeticum), coxsackie virus (eczema coxsackium), or vaccinia virus (eczema vaccinatum) may occur, and treatment should consist of the appropriate antiviral medications, if applicable.[35]

11. **Other important questions/details:**
    a. **What are some common comorbidities associated with AD?**
    AD is associated with various comorbidities, with 50–80% of patients having another atopic or respiratory condition such as food allergy, Wiskott-Aldrich syndrome, allergic rhinitis, or asthma.[1] The risk of developing the atopic triad (AD, allergic rhinitis, and asthma) is inversely associated with the age of onset of AD. Ichthyosis vulgaris is found in 10–30% of patients with AD.[36] Additional associations with this disease include behavioral/psychiatric conditions, such as attention deficit/hyperactivity disorder (ADHD), depression, and anxiety.[37–39]

References

1. Bolognia JL, Schaffer J v, Cerroni L. *Dermatology 2: Volume Set*. 4th ed. Elsevier; 2018.
2. Zackheim HS, McCalmont TH. Mycosis fungoides: The great imitator. *J Am Acad Dermatol*. December, 2002;47(6):914–918.
3. Eichenfield LF, Tom WL, Chamlin SL, et al. Guidelines of care for the management of atopic dermatitis. *J Am Acad Dermatol*. February, 2014;70(2):338–351.
4. Odhiambo JA, Williams HC, Clayton TO, et al. Global variations in prevalence of eczema symptoms in children from ISAAC Phase Three. *J Allergy Clin Immunol*. December, 2009;124(6):1251–8.e23.
5. Williams H, Flohr C. How epidemiology has challenged 3 prevailing concepts about atopic dermatitis. *J Allergy Clin Immunol*. July, 2006;118(1):209–213.
6. Cochran AJ. *McKee's Pathology of the Skin*. Elsevier; 2012.
7. Boguniewicz M, Leung DYM. Atopic dermatitis: A disease of altered skin barrier and immune dysregulation. *Immunol Rev*. July, 2011;242(1):233–246.
8. Mischke D, Korge BP, Marenholz I, Volz A, Ziegler A. Genes encoding structural proteins of epidermal cornification and S100 calcium-binding proteins form a gene complex ("epidermal differentiation complex") on human chromosome 1q21. *J Invest Dermatol*. May, 1996;106(5):989–992.

9. Sandilands A, Sutherland C, Irvine AD, McLean WHI. Filaggrin in the frontline: Role in skin barrier function and disease. *J Cell Sci*. Published online 2009. doi:10.1242/jcs.033969

10. Barnes KC. An update on the genetics of atopic dermatitis: Scratching the surface in 2009. *J Allergy Clin Immunol*. January, 2010;125(1):16–29.e1–11; quiz 30–1.

11. Guttman-Yassky E, Suárez-Fariñas M, Chiricozzi A, et al. Broad defects in epidermal cornification in atopic dermatitis identified through genomic analysis. *J Allergy Clin Immunol*. December, 2009;124(6):1235–1244.e58.

12. Esparza-Gordillo J, Weidinger S, Fölster-Holst R, et al. A common variant on chromosome 11q13 is associated with atopic dermatitis. *Nat Genet*. May, 2009;41(5):596–601.

13. Song SY, Jung SY, Kim EY. Steroid phobia among general users of topical steroids: A cross-sectional nationwide survey. *J Dermatolog Treat*. May, 2019;30(3):245–250.

14. Paternoster L, Standl M, Chen CM, et al. Meta-analysis of genome-wide association studies identifies three new risk loci for atopic dermatitis. *Nat Genet*. December 25, 2011;44(2):187–192.

15. Portelli MA, Hodge E, Sayers I. Genetic risk factors for the development of allergic disease identified by genome-wide association. *Clin Exp Allergy*. January, 2015;45(1):21–31.

16. Broccardo CJ, Mahaffey S, Schwarz J, et al. Comparative proteomic profiling of patients with atopic dermatitis based on history of eczema herpeticum infection and Staphylococcus aureus colonization. *J Allergy Clin Immunol*. January, 2011;127(1):186–193, 193.e1–11.

17. Kuo IH, Yoshida T, de Benedetto A, Beck LA. The cutaneous innate immune response in patients with atopic dermatitis. *J Allergy Clin Immunol*. February, 2013;131(2):266–278.

18. de Benedetto A, Rafaels NM, McGirt LY, et al. Tight junction defects in patients with atopic dermatitis. *J Allergy Clin Immunol*. March, 2011;127(3):773–786.e1–7.

19. de Benedetto A, Agnihothri R, McGirt LY, Bankova LG, Beck LA. Atopic dermatitis: A disease caused by innate immune defects? *J Invest Dermatol*. January, 2009;129(1):14–30.

20. Sokol CL, Barton GM, Farr AG, Medzhitov R. A mechanism for the initiation of allergen-induced T helper type 2 responses. *Nat Immunol*. March, 2008;9(3):310–318.

21. Ziegler SF, Artis D. Sensing the outside world: TSLP regulates barrier immunity. *Nat Immunol*. April, 2010;11(4):289–293.

22. Gao PS, Rafaels NM, Mu D, et al. Genetic variants in thymic stromal lymphopoietin are associated with atopic dermatitis and eczema herpeticum. *J Allergy Clin Immunol*. June, 2010;125(6):1403–1407.e4.

23. Takai T. TSLP expression: Cellular sources, triggers, and regulatory mechanisms. *Allergol Int*. March, 2012;61(1):3–17.

24. Silverman RA. *Hurwitz Clinical Pediatric Dermatology*. 4th ed. Elsevier; 2012.

25. Matiz C, Tom WL, Eichenfield LF, Pong A, Friedlander SF. Children with atopic dermatitis appear less likely to be infected with community acquired methicillin-resistant staphylococcus aureus: The San Diego experience. *Pediatr Dermatol*. January–February, 2011;28(1):6–11.

26. Balma-Mena A, Lara-Corrales I, Zeller J, et al. Colonization with community-acquired methicillin-resistant Staphylococcus aureus in children with atopic dermatitis: A cross-sectional study. *Int J Dermatol*. June, 2011;50(6):682–688.

27. Huang JT, Abrams M, Tlougan B, Rademaker A, Paller AS. Treatment of Staphylococcus aureus colonization in atopic dermatitis decreases disease severity. *Pediatrics*. May, 2009;123(5):e808–e814.

28. Spuls PI, Gerbens LAA, Simpson E, et al. Patient-Oriented Eczema Measure (POEM), a core instrument to measure symptoms in clinical trials: A Harmonising Outcome Measures for Eczema (HOME) statement. *Br J Dermatol*. April, 2017;176(4):979–984.

29. Blauvelt A, Rosmarin D, Bieber T, et al. Improvement of atopic dermatitis with dupilumab occurs equally well across different anatomical regions: Data from phase III clinical trials. *Br J Dermatol*. July, 2019;181(1):196–197.

30. Blauvelt A, de Bruin-Weller M, Gooderham M, et al. Long-term management of moderate-to-severe atopic dermatitis with dupilumab and concomitant topical corticosteroids (LIBERTY AD CHRONOS): A 1-year, randomised, double-blinded, placebo-controlled, phase 3 trial. *Lancet*. June 10, 2017;389(10086):2287–2303.

31. Deleuran M, Thaci D, Beck LA, et al. Dupilumab shows long-term safety and efficacy in patients with moderate to severe atopic dermatitis enrolled in a phase 3 open-label extension study. *J Am Acad Dermatol*. February, 2020;82(2):377–388.

32. Sidbury R, Tom WL, Chamlin SL, et al. Guidelines of care for the management of atopic dermatitis. *J Am Acad Dermatol*. February, 2014;70(2):338–351.

33. Wollenberg A, Barbarot S, Bieber T, et al. Consensus-based European guidelines for treatment of atopic eczema (atopic dermatitis) in adults and children: Part I. *J Eur Acad Dermatol Venereol*. May, 2018;32(5):657–682.

34. Reynolds NJ, Franklin V, Gray JC, Diffey BL, Farr PM. Narrow-band ultraviolet B and broad-band ultraviolet a phototherapy in adult atopic eczema: A randomised controlled trial. *Lancet*. June 23, 2001;357(9273):2012–2016.

35. Mohan GC, Lio PA. Comparison of dermatology and allergy guidelines for atopic dermatitis management. *JAMA Dermatol*. September, 2015;151(9):1009–1013.

36. Bremmer SF, Hanifin JM, Simpson EL. Clinical detection of ichthyosis vulgaris in an atopic dermatitis clinic: Implications for allergic respiratory disease and prognosis. *J Am Acad Dermatol*. July, 2008;59(1):72–78.

37. Yaghmaie P, Koudelka CW, Simpson EL. Mental health comorbidity in patients with atopic dermatitis. *J Allergy Clin Immunol*. February, 2013;131(2):428–433.

38. Patel KR, Immaneni S, Singam V, Rastogi S, Silverberg JI. Association between atopic dermatitis, depression, and suicidal ideation: A systematic review and meta-analysis. *J Am Acad Dermatol*. February, 2019;80(2):402–410.

39. Thyssen JP, Hamann CR, Linneberg A, et al. Atopic dermatitis is associated with anxiety, depression, and suicidal ideation, but not with psychiatric hospitalization or suicide. *Allergy*. January, 2018;73(1):214–220.

40. Feldman SR, Cox LS, Strowd LC, et al. The challenge of managing atopic dermatitis in the United States. *Am Heal Drug Benefits*. April, 2019;12(2):83–93.

4

Soft, Subcutaneous Nodule with Central Dark Punctum

JALAL MAGHFOUR AND CRISTIAN C. RIVIS

A 21-year-old male presents to the clinic for a nodule on the right side of his neck, which he first noticed several months ago (Figure 4.1). He denies any pruritus, bleeding, pain, or change in the size of the lesion. The lesion is not bothersome; however, the patient has noticed an occasional foul-smelling, thick, white discharge. He has not attempted any treatments and denies any exacerbating or alleviating factors. Family history is positive for malignant melanoma. The patient is otherwise healthy.

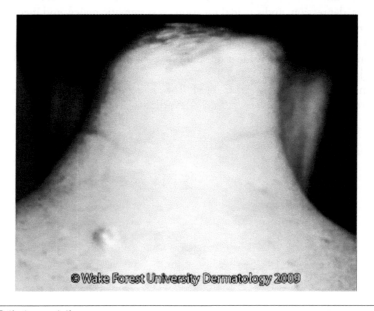

Figure 4.1   Patient presentation.

1. **How would you describe the lesion?**
   The lesion is a 1.0-cm, skin-colored, soft, deep dermal-to-subcutaneous nodule with an overlying central dark punctum.

 DOI: 10.1201/9781003437987-4

2. What are the differential diagnoses (Table 4.1)?

Table 4.1   Differential Diagnoses for a Soft, Subcutaneous Nodule with a Central Dark Punctum

DIAGNOSIS	COMMENTS
Lipoma	A lipoma is a common benign tumor of mature adipocytes. Lipomas are usually asymptomatic and affect middle-aged individuals (men more than women) but can manifest at any age. A lipoma is described as a soft to rubbery, occasionally multilobular, and mobile subcutaneous nodule with a normal overlying epidermis. Risk factors include diabetes, obesity, and hypercholesterolemia.[1]
Pilar cyst	Also known as trichilemmal cysts. A pilar cyst is a common dermal entity that arises from the isthmus of the follicular canal. It often affects middle-aged individuals (women more than men). Clinically, these cysts present as a solitary lesion with a predilection for the scalp. Pilar cysts appear in a sporadic manner but may be inherited as an autosomal dominant trait.[2]
Pilomatricoma	Also known as pilomatrixoma. A pilomatricoma is a benign tumor of hair follicles that accounts for less than 1% of all benign cutaneous neoplasms. The majority of cases arise in childhood and adolescence. A pilomatricoma presents as a solitary, asymptomatic, skin-colored or blue lesion.[3]
Steatocystoma multiplex	A steatocystoma is a cystic lesion that arises from the dermis. It is a rare entity that affects men and women equally. Clinically, steatocystoma multiplex can manifest as asymptomatic, skin-colored to yellow nodules with a predilection for the chest, axillae, and groin; it is unusual for these lesions to develop on the head and neck region. Unlike the characteristic thick white discharge seen with epidermoid cysts, an oil-like fluid may be drained from steatocystoma multiplex lesions.[2]
Epidermoid cyst	Epidermoid cysts are nodular masses with clearly defined borders that may be as small as a few millimeters and can grow to several centimeters in diameter. They often develop from infundibular dysfunction within a follicle that accumulates keratin within an expanding cavity. These nodules may range in color from skin-toned to a yellowish hue. Often a dark punctum at the location of the causative impacted follicle may be present over the mass and may aid in diagnosis. Although cysts usually remain asymptomatic, they may become inflamed and rupture, which may release foul-smelling drainage and cause significant pain. Epidermoid cysts most commonly present on the head, neck, and upper torso but can occur on any skin surface, albeit less frequently.[4]

3. What is the most likely diagnosis?

The most likely diagnosis for this patient is an epidermoid cyst.

4. What is the next best step?

The next best step in management for a clinically stable, non-inflamed epidermoid cyst is observation and reassurance due to the benign nature of the lesion. While family history of malignant melanoma is concerning, various factors favor a benign process in this patient, including a slow rate of growth; thick, white discharge; and lack of pigmentation in addition to the morphologic features that characterize an epidermoid cyst lesion. Thus, a biopsy is unnecessary.

5. What are the most appropriate diagnostic modalities (i.e., labs, biopsies, scrapings, histological findings)?

Epidermoid cysts are a clinical diagnosis that require evaluation based on a history and physical examination alone. However, the diagnosis can also be confirmed via incision and drainage of the lesion, which will reveal a foul-smelling, thick, white discharge. Biopsy for histological and pathological results is unnecessary even for epidermoid cysts that require surgical excision.[4]

6. **What would you expect to find in the histopathologic analysis?**

   The histological examination will reveal an enclosed cyst filled with laminated keratinous material and lined by a stratified squamous epithelium that contains a granular layer. If the cyst ruptures, keratin granuloma and fibrosis can be seen as a result of an acute and chronic inflammatory process. In human papillomavirus (HPV)–infected epidermoid cysts, the epithelium demonstrates acanthosis with a verrucous cyst wall appearance.[4]

7. **Discuss the epidemiology of this disease**.

   a. **Discuss the incidence and prevalence:**

      Epidermoid cysts are common benign lesions and tend to affect men more than women, with a ratio of 2:1, and no racial predilection. While epidermoid cysts commonly affect younger individuals as well as those in their third and fourth decades of life, they rarely appear before puberty. The exact incidence remains unknown, as these lesions are common and are infrequently brought to a physician's attention unless a patient is concerned for a malignancy, such as in this case of a symptomatic ruptured epidermoid cyst.[4] Although epidermoid cysts are highly prevalent, malignant transformation into squamous cell carcinoma (SCC) and basal cell carcinoma (BCC) is rare, with an incidence of about 1 in 3,000.[5]

   b. **Discuss the sociodemographics of individuals affected by this disease (i.e., age, gender, race, geographic location, other risk factors):**

      Higher-risk individuals include men and elderly individuals with chronic sun damage due to skin atrophy and keratinization of pilosebaceous follicles secondary to prolonged ultraviolet exposure (Table 4.2).[4]

Table 4.2   Risk Factors Associated with Epidermoid Cysts

RISK FACTOR	COMMENTS
Gender	Men are more commonly affected than women, with a ratio of 2:1.[4]
Age	Middle-aged and elderly individuals with a history of chronic sun damage are at increased risk.[6]
Human papillomavirus (HPV) infection	HPV 60 is implicated in the development of palmoplantar epidermoid cysts.[4]
Iatrogenic/traumatic implantation	Deep penetrating injuries cause implantation of epidermal elements into the dermis.[4]

Since epidermoid cysts originate from the follicular infundibulum, conditions that result in the disruption of the follicle, such as acne vulgaris, can precipitate their formation. Small epidermoid cysts, also known as milia, are common during the neonatal period. Most cases of epidermoid cysts arise sporadically but may be genetically linked. This is seen in the setting of Gardner syndrome, basal cell nevus syndrome (Gorlin syndrome), and Favre-Racouchot syndrome (Table 4.3).[6]

Table 4.3 Genetic Syndromes Associated with Epidermoid Cysts

GENETIC SYNDROME	COMMENTS
Basal cell nevus syndrome (Gorlin syndrome)	A rare disorder inherited in an autosomal dominant pattern. Prevalence in the United States is estimated to be between 1 in 31,000 and 1 in 164,000. The majority of cases are due to a *PTCH1* gene mutation, as *PTCH1* plays an important role in cellular signaling. The hallmark of this disorder is the occurrence of multiple basal cell carcinomas (BCCs) around the age of puberty.[7] Epidermoid cysts are a known manifestation of this syndrome and tend to present in multiples before puberty. Epidermoid cysts may present in unusual regions, including the face and extremities.[4]
Favre-Racouchot syndrome	This is a benign, non-hereditary disorder that is also known as solar or senile comedones, or nodular elastosis with cysts and comedones. It affects approximately less than 10% of the U.S. population with a predilection for middle-aged Caucasian men. Risk factors include a history of smoking and previous exposure to radiation.[8] The hallmark of this syndrome is the presence of multiple open comedones and epidermoid cysts on a background of sun-damaged skin. Lesions often appear on the cheeks, temples, and periorbital regions. In these individuals, epidermoid cysts are believed to develop secondary to chronic ultraviolet light exposure.[8]
Gardner syndrome	Gardner syndrome is an autosomal dominant variant of familial adenomatous polyposis (FAP). In the United States, the prevalence is estimated to be 1 per 1 million.[9] In addition to colonic polyposis, extracutaneous manifestations are commonly reported in Gardner syndrome. Fifty to sixty percent of patients develop epidermoid cysts, the most common extracolonic manifestation. Similarly to Gorlin syndrome, epidermoid cysts tend to appear before puberty and in unusual locations such as on the face, scalp, and extremities.

Recent studies identify HPV infection as a risk factor in the pathogenesis of epidermoid cyst formation. The exact mechanism remains unknown. However, in rare instances, epidermoid cysts can develop on the soles, which has been associated with HPV 60 infection.[10,11]

8. **Discuss the pathogenesis of this disease.**

The pathogenesis of epidermoid cysts can be divided into primary and secondary etiology. A primary process entails the development of an epidermoid cyst directly from the infundibulum of a hair follicle. This is due to the plugging of the follicular orifice leading to cyst formation. This is often the process by which patients with acne vulgaris can develop such lesions from pre-existing comedones, as the blockage of pores and the disruption of hair follicles increase the risk of epidermoid cyst development.[6] A secondary process refers to the implantation and proliferation of follicular epithelium into the dermis due to trauma. Secondary processes often take place in surface areas denuded of hair follicles such as on the palms and soles.[4]

9. **What is the clinical presentation of this disease (i.e., grade, stage, subtypes)?**

Clinically, non-inflamed epidermoid cysts are asymptomatic. They appear as dome-shaped, firm, skin-colored nodules that are freely mobile upon palpation; oftentimes, a central dilated punctum can be appreciated.[4] On the other hand, ruptured epidermoid cysts are painful upon palpation and appear erythematous and fluctuant, mimicking an abscess. Following the acute inflammatory process, a ruptured epidermoid cyst may also induce foreign body reaction, leading to granuloma formation. Such epidermoid cysts become adherent to the surrounding tissue and clinically present as a hard, immobile mass, which makes them difficult to excise.[6]

10. **Discuss treatment options.**

Epidermoid cyst treatment options may vary based on the degree of inflammation. For non-inflamed asymptomatic epidermoid cysts, treatment is not necessary. Most epidermoid cysts reach a stable size, often in the range of a few millimeters to centimeters. For patients desiring cyst removal for cosmetic reasons, surgical excision may be performed if the cyst is not inflamed. This is accomplished by incising the skin overlying the cyst, which expresses the cyst contents, followed by a blunt dissection of the cyst and its wall. The cyst wall, in its entirety, must be removed in order to prevent recurrence. All surgically excised epidermoid cysts are sent for histopathological confirmation.[4] If a cyst ruptures during excision, a curette may be used to remove the remaining cyst contents and wall. In a cyst that has previously ruptured and subsequently scarred, an elliptical excision is required.[7]

In the setting of an inflamed cyst, surgical and medical intervention is required, as inflamed cysts rarely resolve without treatment. An inflamed cyst is treated as an abscess, requiring incision and drainage. Occasionally, a course of antibiotics is provided; however, cultures from fluid collected often yield negative results. Use of intralesional corticosteroids can hasten the inflammatory process and provide symptomatic relief.[7]

References

1. Kaddu S. Smooth muscle, adipose and cartilage neoplasms. In: Bolognia J, Schaffer JV, Lorenzo C, eds. *Dermatology*. 4th ed. Elsevier; 2018:2086–2101.
2. Al Aboud DM, Patel BC. Pilar cyst. In: *StatPearls*. Treasure Island, FL: StatPearls Publishing LLC.; 2020.
3. Julian CG, Bowers PW. A clinical review of 209 pilomatricomas. *J Am Acad Dermatol*. 1998;39(2 Pt 1):191–195.
4. Stone M. Cysts In: Bolognia J, Schaffer JV, Lorenzo C, eds. *Dermatology*. 4th ed. Elsevier; 2018:1917–1929.
5. Faltaous AA, Leigh EC, Ray P, Wolbert TT. A rare transformation of epidermoid cyst into squamous cell carcinoma: A case report with literature review. *Am J Case Rep*. 2019;20:1141–1143.

6. Ramagosa R, de Villiers EM, Fitzpatrick JE, Dellavalle RP. Human papillomavirus infection and ultraviolet light exposure as epidermoid inclusion cyst risk factors in a patient with epidermodysplasia verruciformis? *J Am Acad Dermatol.* 2008;58(5 Suppl 1):S68.e61–66.
7. James WD, Elston DM, Treat JR, Rosenbach M, Neuhaus I. Epidermal nevi, neoplasms, and cysts. In: James WD, Elston DM, Treat JR, Rosenbach M, Neuhaus I, eds. *Andrews' Diseases of the Skin: Clinical Dermatology.* 13th ed. Elsevier; 2020:636–685.
8. Fujii K, Miyashita T. Gorlin syndrome (nevoid basal cell carcinoma syndrome): Update and literature review. *Pediatr Int.* 2014;56(5):667–674.
9. Patterson WM, Fox MD, Schwartz RA. Favre-Racouchot disease. *Int J Dermatol.* 2004;43(3):167–169.
10. Lewis KG, Bercovitch L, Dill SW, Robinson-Bostom L. Acquired disorders of elastic tissue: Part I. Increased elastic tissue and solar elastotic syndromes. *J Am Acad Dermatol.* 2004;51(1):1–21; quiz 22–24.
11. Juhn E, Khachemoune A. Gardner syndrome: Skin manifestations, differential diagnosis and management. *Am J Clin Dermatol.* 2010;11(2):117–122.

5

ASYMMETRIC, BROWN TO BLACK VARIEGATED MACULE WITH IRREGULAR BORDERS

JARETT CASALE AND CRISTIAN C. RIVIS

A 58-year-old female with a history of multiple severe, blistering sunburns as a teenager presents with an 8-mm, dark brown macule on her left cheek that has increased in size over the past 2 years (Figure 5.1). She denies bleeding but notes intermittent pruritus. The patient has multiple characteristic light brown nevi with regular borders on her lower extremities bilaterally, all less than 5 mm.

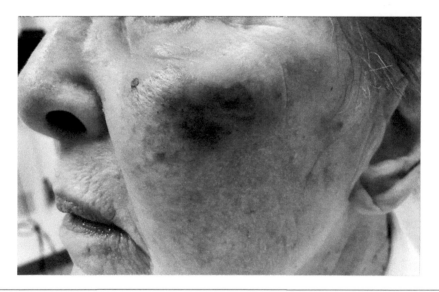

Figure 5.1 Patient presentation.

1. **How would you describe the lesion?**

   The lesion on her cheek is an asymmetric, 8-mm, light brown to black variegated macule with irregular borders.

DOI: 10.1201/9781003437987-5

2. What are the differential diagnoses (Table 5.1)?

Table 5.1 Differential Diagnoses for Asymmetric Brown to Black Variegated Macules with Irregular Borders

DIAGNOSIS	COMMENTS
Atypical nevus	Can possess many characteristics alarming for malignancy, including dark and irregular pigmentation and indistinct or irregular borders. Such nevi are often greater than 5–10 mm, with new lesions continuing to appear even after age 40. Atypical nevi do not typically demonstrate rapid progression in size.[1]
Blue nevus	Blue nevi contain a dark pigment network that is uniformly distributed. Depositions of excess pigment in the dermis are responsible for the bluish color observed. These nevi are typically dome-shaped papules less than 5 mm in diameter and have round and regular margins.[1]
Melanoma	Vary greatly in clinical features, but typically contain an irregular pigment network with color variegation and irregular borders that evolve over time. The lesion may change in color as it progresses, with sudden darkening; appearance of red, blue, or white coloration; and invasion into healthy skin. The development of a halo of depigmentation around the lesion, changes in the shape of the border, and the appearance of pigment satellites are developments that are suspicious for melanoma in adults. Melanoma lesions may also bleed, scale, ulcerate, ooze, or form crusts.[1]
Pigmented basal cell carcinoma (BCC)	BCCs may present as a lesion with brown to bluish gray to black pigmentation. They are often identified as having a white, translucent, and elevated border. Arborizing telangiectasias, blue-gray ovoid nests, and ulcerations may also be noted upon close visual examination.[1]
Pigmented squamous cell carcinoma (SCC)	Pigmented SCCs present as nodular or papular, erythematous or pigmented lesions. Biopsies are helpful to identify horned pearls along with melanocytes and atypical epidermal squamous cells.[2]

3. What is the most likely diagnosis?

The most likely diagnosis for this patient is a superficial spreading malignant melanoma.

4. What is the next best step?

The next best step in the management of this lesion with a high degree of clinical suspicion for melanoma is excision in toto, or removal of the entire lesion, including the epidermis, dermis, and subcutaneous adipose tissue with 1- to 2-mm margins.[3] The method of biopsy obtained for pigmented lesions depends on the degree of clinical suspicion for melanoma. For pigmented lesions that do not meet all the ABCDE criteria (*A*symmetry, *B*order irregularity, *C*olor variation, *D*iameter greater than 6 mm, and *E*volving characteristics) but are concerning for atypia, a shave biopsy that removes the entirety of the pigmented lesion may be preferred. After the preferred method of biopsy is performed, clinical re-evaluation of the biopsy area and specimen should take place to ensure that the margins of pigment have been excised in entirety. If any pigment surrounding the initial lesion remains, it is imperative to excise the remaining pigment to ensure clear margins for an accurate pathological and histological diagnosis.[3]

5. What are the most appropriate diagnostic modalities (i.e., labs, biopsies, scrapings, histological findings)?

Melanoma is diagnosed by a combination of clinical and histological findings. The clinical workup for melanoma should include consideration of the ABCDE criteria and the "ugly duckling" sign (Table 5.2).[1] The "ugly duckling" sign describes a lesion that stands out from the rest of the patient's characteristic nevi.[3] This sign should be considered for atypical nevi even if they do not fulfill all the ABCDE criteria.

Table 5.2   ABCDE Criteria Suspicious for Melanoma

CRITERION	DESCRIPTION
Asymmetry	One half of the mole does not match the other.
Borders	The edges are irregular, ragged, notched, or blurred.
Color	The mole is unevenly colored; it may have variations of brown or black, patches of pink, red, white, or blue.
Diameter	The mole is larger than 6 mm in diameter.
Evolving	The mole is changing in size, shape, or color.

The use of dermoscopy, or skin surface microscopy, is often helpful in recognizing lesion criteria that can aid in the diagnosis of melanoma. These criteria include categories of global and local features (Table 5.3). Global features of melanoma on dermoscopy include color variegation, or the presence of multiple colors within a suspected lesion. Local features of dermoscopy suspicious for melanoma include a blue-white veil, atypical network, streaks, irregular blood vessels, and regression structures. Lastly, patterns seen in melanoma commonly have multiple components consisting of three or more patterns within one lesion.[3]

Table 5.3   Global and Local Features Suspicious for Melanoma

GLOBAL FEATURES	LOCAL FEATURES
• Multicomponent pattern (three or more patterns) • Unspecific pattern (structureless or two irregular patterns) • Parallel pattern (along ridges; palms and soles only)	• Atypical pigment network (branched, broken up, thickened, asymmetrical) • Irregularly distributed dots/globules of different sizes and shapes • Asymmetrical blotches • Five or six colors (black, brown, tan, gray, blue, red, white) • Blue-white veil • White, scar-like depigmentation • Blue pepper-like granules • On face: gray dots, pseudo-network, rhomboidal structures, asymmetrical pigmented follicles, annular-granular structures

Following excisional biopsy, the gold standard for the diagnosis of melanoma is histopathological analysis. Mandatory components of the histopathologic report for melanoma include a diagnosis of malignant melanoma, tumor thickness, presence of ulceration, and margins. Desirable components of the histopathologic report include the histopathologic subtype of melanoma, presence of plasma cells or lymphocytes, vascular invasion, microscopic satellites, and mitotic rate. The depth of invasion of malignant melanoma is the major prognostic factor and predictor of survival and is known as Breslow depth. In addition to depth of invasion, several histological features should be noted to determine the prognosis. For cases in which the histopathological findings for melanoma are equivocal, immunohistochemical studies can be used to aid in diagnosis. Commonly used immunohistochemical stains for diagnosis include HMB45, tyrosinase, MART-1, and S100 antigens. Definitive diagnosis of melanoma includes a workup that involves tumor staging.[3]

6. **What would you expect to find in the histopathologic analysis?**

   The lesion in the clinical vignette is most likely a superficial spreading melanoma. Histopathologic features of superficial spreading melanoma include irregular intraepidermal nests and complexes of atypical lymphocytes present in the dermis. The atypical melanocytes are noted to have prominent nucleoli.[3]

7. **Discuss the epidemiology of this disease**.

   a. **Discuss the incidence and prevalence:**

      Melanoma is the most rapidly increasing skin cancer in Caucasians.[3,4] It represents the fifth most common cancer in men and sixth most common cancer in women.[1] This increase in incidence is evidenced by a rise from 8.2:9.4 (female:male) cases per 100,000 in 1975 to 24.2:35.4 (female:male) cases per 100,000 in 2010.[5] The current lifetime risk of developing melanoma for Americans today is 1 in 63, compared to 1 in 1,500 in 1935.[1]

   b. **Discuss the sociodemographics of individuals affected by this disease (i.e., age, gender, race, geographic location, other risk factors):**

      Melanoma is typically diagnosed in older individuals, with a median age of diagnosis at 57 years old. Males have a 1.5 times increased risk for developing melanoma compared to females. Melanoma is most prevalent in the Caucasian population, at a 10 times greater risk than African American or Hispanic individuals. Melanoma has a geographic predilection for regions with increased sun exposure; Australia and New Zealand have the highest incidence.[1] Risk for the development of melanoma in an individual results from the interaction between host factors, genetic factors, and sun exposure. The main environmental risk factor for melanoma is sun exposure, which can be divided into three categories: intermittent, chronic, and total exposure. Intermittent exposure includes short, intense exposures typically followed by sunburn. Chronic exposure describes continuous exposure that is primarily occupational. Total sun exposure is the sum of intermittent and chronic exposure. The strongest association for melanoma risk results from the intermittent pattern of sun exposure. Total exposure also exhibits a positive association with melanoma risk.[5] In addition to sun exposure, ultraviolet (UV) exposure from tanning beds is a major risk factor in the development of melanoma. Genetic factors play a role in melanoma development. For example, 40% of members of melanoma-prone families have germline mutations in the tumor suppressor gene cyclin-dependent kinase inhibitor 2A (*CDKN2A*).[4] Other risk factors for melanoma development include type and number of nevi. Individuals with more than 100 normal nevi are at nearly seven times greater risk for melanoma than individuals with fewer than 15 normal nevi.[5]

8. **Discuss the pathogenesis of this disease**.

Melanoma, like all malignancies, results from aberrations in genetic signaling that lead to uninhibited cellular proliferation and evasion of apoptosis. This typically occurs due to genetic mutations that result in overactivation of proto-oncogenes or inactivation of tumor suppressor genes, or a combination of both. In melanoma, the primary dysfunctional cellular signaling pathway depends on the source of genetic damage. For example, melanomas arising in intermittently sun-damaged skin are more likely to carry a mutation in the proto-oncogene *BRAF* as compared with melanomas present in chronically sun-damaged skin. Melanomas arising from chronically sun-damaged skin are more likely to contain UV-signature mutations. *BRAF* mutations are found in 44–70% of melanomas, and most of these cases contain a genetic alteration leading to a substitution at codon 600 of glutamic acid (E) for valine (V), known as a V600E mutation. This mutation leads to activation of the mitogen-activated protein kinase (MAPK) pathway.[1]

MAPK is one of the most studied cellular pathways involved in melanoma and is heavily involved in cellular proliferation and migration.[5] Genes that encode for the components of MAPK include *BRAF*, *NRAS*, and *CDK2NA*. Mutations of the *CDKN2A* gene can predispose individuals to familial melanoma. In addition to the MAPK pathway, activation of phosphoinositide 3-kinases (PI3Ks) are implicated in many melanomas through inactivation of the tumor suppressor phosphatase and tensin homolog (PTEN) or activation of the proto-oncogene *NRAS*. In addition to the mentioned signaling pathways, many more processes have been identified in the pathogenesis and progression of melanoma. The advent of genetic testing in the treatment of melanoma has allowed for a more specific and targeted approach to treatment.[3]

9. **What is the clinical presentation of this disease (i.e., grade, stage, subtypes)?**

The most common early symptoms leading to clinical presentation may include an increase in lesion size, a change in the color or shape of the lesion, and pruritus. However, most lesions are completely asymptomatic. The clinical appearance of melanoma varies significantly, and no single color or change is diagnostic. Melanoma can develop de novo or within a pre-existing lesion.

The most common subtype, superficial spreading melanoma, may arise within a pre-existing lesion about 50% of the time.[3]

There are four major subtypes of melanoma: superficial spreading, nodular, lentigo maligna, and acral lentiginous (Table 5.4).

Table 5.4   Major Subtypes of Melanoma

MELANOMA SUBTYPE	PERCENTAGE OF TOTAL CASES	MOST COMMON SITE(S)	DESCRIPTION
Superficial spreading	60–70%[1]	• Upper back (both men and women) • Legs (women)[1]	• Asymmetric, irregularly bordered macule or papule with or without color variegation. • Often diagnosed when <5 mm but can grow to be significantly larger. • Preference for radial (horizontal) growth of melanocytic proliferation, most commonly limited to the epidermis.[5]
Nodular	15–20%[1]	• Trunk • Legs[1]	• Variants include spitzoid melanoma, atypical fibroxanthoma-like melanoma, and collision tumors. • Preference for vertical growth of melanocytic proliferation and is therefore typically diagnosed at a deeper, more advanced stage.[5]
Lentigo maligna	4–15%[1]	• Head • Neck • Arms[1]	• Flat, irregularly outlined lesion with irregular pigment network that extends beyond the clinical lesion. • Typically seen in chronically sun-damaged individuals. • Unlike superficial spreading melanoma, lentigo maligna melanoma is unrelated to nevus count. • Less aggressive, with 5% progressing to invasive melanoma.[3]
Acral lentiginous	~5%; up to 70% in African Americans; up to 45% in Asians[3]	• Palms • Soles • Nail beds	• Asymmetric brown-to-black macule with color variegation. • When involving the proximal nail body, may present with longitudinal melanonychia (Hutchinson's sign).[5]

Melanoma is staged by the American Joint Committee on Cancer (AJCC) system from 0 to IV depending on the extent of invasion and metastasis (Table 5.5). The AJCC stage is determined by a combination of the Tumor-Node-Metastases (TNM) classification system. The clinical staging system for melanoma also includes subcategories of the TNM system, including microstaging of the primary melanoma as well as radiologic and clinical metastatic evaluation. Tumor (T) refers to the tumor thickness (Breslow depth) and presence of ulceration of the primary lesion. Node (N) refers to the extent of regional lymph node metastases and separates stage III from stages I and II. Metastasis (M) refers to detection of distant metastases beyond regional lymph nodes and indicates stage IV.[3]

Table 5.5   Staging Characteristics of Melanoma

AJCC STAGE[a]	CLINICAL STAGING	THICKNESS (MM)	ULCERATION	METASTASIS	5-YEAR SURVIVAL (%) (BALCH ET AL.)
0		T_{IS}[b]	In situ	–	–	NA
I	IA	T1a	<0.8	–	–	97
	IB	T1b	<0.8	Yes	–	93
		T1b	0.8–1.0	–	–	93
		T2a	1.0–2.0	–	–	93
II	IIA	T2b	1.0–2.0	Yes	–	82
		T3a	2.0–4.0	–	–	79
	IIB	T3b	2.0–4.0	Yes	–	68
		T4a	>4.0	–	–	71
	IIC	T4b	>4.0	Yes	–	53
III	IIIA—IIID	Any T or T_{IS} with N			Regional nodal/ lymphatic metastasis	40–78
IV	IV	Any T or N with M			Distant metastasis	9–27

[a] AJCC stage is based on a combination of T, N, M classification. Clinical stage includes T, N, M subcategories determined by the microstage of the primary tumor (T), including tumor thickness (Breslow depth) and presence/absence of ulceration, combined with presence of lymph node (N) metastasis or distant metastasis (M).
[b] Melanoma in situ is defined by confinement of malignant cells above the epidermal basement membrane.[1]

AJCC: American Joint Committee on Cancer; **IS:** in situ; **N:** lymph node; **NA:** not applicable; **T:** tumor

10. Discuss treatment options.

Melanoma management options depend on the stage and severity of the subtype involved. For primary cutaneous melanoma (stages 0–II), surgical excision with margins is the mainstay of treatment. The size of the surgical margin taken is based on the tumor thickness. Management of melanoma in situ (malignant cells confined to the epidermis), includes wide excision with 0.5- to 1.0-cm margins.[1] For stage I tumors with Breslow depth <1 mm, current guidelines state that a safety margin of 1 cm is sufficient for preventing tumor recurrence. For melanomas of Breslow depth 1–4 mm, current guidelines recommend a 2-cm safety margin.[3] Recommendations for surgical excision include excising to the depth of muscle fascia, if possible, given the anatomic location.[1] Surgical management of melanomas present in an anatomical area not conducive to safety margins, such as the face, may include the use of Mohs micrographic surgery.[3] When surgical management is not clinically feasible, non-surgical options may be considered including topical imiquimod, cryosurgery, and radiation therapy.[1]

For melanoma with Breslow depth greater than 1 mm, sentinel lymph node biopsy is performed to determine the extent of invasion into surrounding lymph nodes. Sentinel lymph node status is a major prognostic factor for overall survival and recurrence of melanoma.[3] If metastasis is found to be present in surrounding lymph nodes, patients can be offered adjuvant systemic therapy with various agents, including interferon-α (IFN-α) or monoclonal antibodies such as vemurafenib (selective *BRAF* inhibitor) and ipilimumab (monoclonal antibody against cytotoxic T-lymphocyte antigen 4 [CTLA-4]). In patients with a V600E *BRAF* mutation, the use of vemurafenib prolongs overall survival. Ipilimumab also prolongs overall survival in patients with distant metastatic disease.[1] For advanced cases with distant metastasis (stage IV), kinase inhibitors have been used with moderate success, although development of drug resistance remains an ongoing issue. Surgical resection of distant metastases helps palliatively and promotes long-term survival in some patients.[3,4]

11. **Other important questions/details:**
How to reduce risk for development of melanoma
Sun protection is a primary preventative practice to reduce the risk of developing melanoma. Sun protective clothing and the use of hats provide more sun protection than the use of chemical sunscreens.[1] Limiting outdoor activities during hours of peak sun intensity (10 am–2 pm) should also be practiced. Regular sunscreen use should not provide a false sense of security from photodamage. Repeated ultraviolet (UV) exposure at levels low enough to avoid sunburn can induce DNA damage that can eventually lead to skin cancer.[3]

Follow-up after diagnosis of melanoma
Following diagnosis and treatment of malignant melanoma, patients should undergo routine total body skin examinations, including lymph node palpation, every 3–12 months indefinitely based on provider discretion. Routine laboratory surveillance tests for evaluation of metastasis are not currently recommended in patients with a history of melanoma due to high false-positive rates.[6]

Immunological response to melanoma
Clinical evidence of rare instances of spontaneous melanoma regression followed by depigmentation and fibrosis points to the recognition of melanoma cells by the host immune system. Recognition of various melanoma antigens by CD8+ cytotoxic T cells, as well as host antibodies, plays a role in tumor regression. As tumor cells become more advanced, their ability to evade host immunity increases. Research on the interplay of the host immune system

with melanoma is a promising field that may lead to more effective treatments for melanoma in the future.[3]

Amelanotic melanoma

Amelanotic melanoma is a rare subtype of melanoma but should be considered on the differential diagnosis of a clinically suspicious lesion. Amelanotic refers to a melanoma that lacks the characteristic pigmentation of melanoma, making diagnosis particularly difficult. Lesions can present as skin-colored or light pink in color, and the degree of clinical suspicion should guide the need for a biopsy. Amelanotic variants can be seen in any of the four major subtypes of melanoma and are identical in prognosis and therapeutic approach.[3]

References

1. Habif TP. *Clinical Dermatology*. 6th ed. China: Elsevier; 2016.
2. Morais PM, Schettini APM, Rocha JA, Silva Júnior RCD. Pigmented squamous cell carcinoma: Case report and importance of differential diagnosis. *An Bras Dermatol*. 2018;93(1):96–98.
3. Bolognia J, Lorenzo C, Shaffer JV. *Dermatology*. 4th ed. Elsevier; 2018.
4. Bosserhoff A. *Melanoma Development*. New York: Springer; 2011.
5. Kaufman HL, Mehnert JM. *Melanoma*. Vol 167. Switzerland: Springer International Publishing; 2016.
6. Bichakjian CK, Halpern AC, Johnson TM, et al. Guidelines of care for the management of primary cutaneous melanoma: American Academy of Dermatology. *J Am Acad Dermatol*. 2011;65(5):1032–1047.

6

ERYTHEMATOUS, EXCORIATED, PRURITIC PAPULES

SAIRA KHAN AND CRISTIAN C. RIVIS

A 2-year-old male with no significant past medical history presents to the clinic with a 1-day history of itching and "rash" over the bilateral lower extremities (Figure 6.1). The patient's mother noticed the rash last night after they returned from an outdoor barbeque. She observed him scratching toward the end of the barbeque, but she did not notice any rash at that time. The following morning his mother noticed several distinct areas of redness surrounding a central raised point. The patient wore a long-sleeved shirt and shorts when he attended the barbeque. He has had prior similar episodes when spending time outside during the warmer months. His mother did not apply any topical treatment to his legs and has not given him any oral medications. She denies that he has any medication or food allergies. He has not been given any new products and has not had any fever or recent infections.

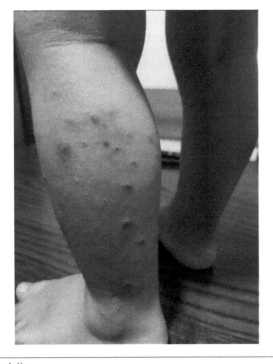

Figure 6.1 Patient presentation.

DOI: 10.1201/9781003437987-6

1. How would you describe the lesion?

The lesions are diffusely scattered over the bilateral lower legs, sparing the feet, and have a papular urticarial appearance. The lesions are discrete and measure 5–8 mm in diameter. Each lesion has a central papule with an area of surrounding erythema, and many lesions are excoriated. The lesions are nontender to palpation, and there is no evidence of discharge.

2. What are the differential diagnoses (Table 6.1)?

Table 6.1   Differential Diagnoses for Erythematous, Excoriated, Pruritic Papules

DIAGNOSIS	COMMENTS
Urticaria	Urticaria, or hives, is an immune-mediated reaction (most commonly IgE-mediated) that is characterized by the acute onset of intense pruritus and transient wheals on the skin that rapidly change in appearance and location on the body. Urticaria can be brought on by recent upper respiratory tract infections (mostly in children), ingestion of certain drugs or foods, recent aspirin or NSAID use, stress, physical exercise, sunlight, heat, cold, and pressure.[1]
Bedbug bites	Bedbug bites (*Cimex lectularius*) can present as papular urticaria over exposed skin areas; however, they typically appear as papules in groups of three. This is known as the "breakfast, lunch, and dinner" pattern. The patient may also describe reddish-brown streaks on their sheets or mattress, which represent where the bedbugs defecate their blood meals.[2]
Cellulitis	Cellulitis is an infection of the skin, most commonly caused by group A streptococci or *Staphylococcus aureus*, that presents as a localized area of erythema and warmth. It often presents in the lower extremities in adults; however, it is typically unilateral. Cellulitis tends to be painful to touch and often spreads over a larger area as the infection progresses. Cellulitis is also frequently accompanied by a fever.[1]
Allergic contact dermatitis	Allergic contact dermatitis is a type IV delayed hypersensitivity reaction (HSR) that is cell-mediated in nature. It typically arises from contact with a hapten, a small immunogenic molecule capable of combining with proteins on the surface of epidermal macrophages. This hapten-protein complex stimulates the formation of lymphocytes against the allergen, and when the host is re-exposed to the same antigen, these lymphocytes elicit an immune response 1–2 days after re-exposure.[1] The HSR that follows is erythematous and typically appears as either sharply demarcated patches or plaques or linear papulovesicles (more common with poison ivy or poison oak exposure).[1,2] While the presentation may vary, it almost always occurs in skin that was in direct contact with the allergen.
Insect bite reaction	An insect bite reaction caused by an arthropod can produce papular urticaria, typically after outdoor exposure in a warm, humid climate.[3,4] While the pain of an insect sting is usually felt immediately, insect bites—especially those of mosquitoes—are often not felt when they occur.[1] The erythematous, urticarial papules can measure 2–8 mm and are often excoriated if the patient has intense pruritus in the areas of the bites.[3] There is often a central punctum.[1] Bite reactions can be urticarial, eczematous, bullous, or granulomatous.[1,2,5] The bite reactions may be disseminated or grouped and usually appear in areas of the body that were exposed to the insect.[3]

NSAID: nonsteroidal anti-inflammatory drug; **HSR:** hypersensitivity reaction

3. What is the most likely diagnosis?

Given this patient's history of recent outdoor exposure and characteristic physical exam findings, the most likely diagnosis is multiple insect bites, specifically mosquito bites.

4. **What is the next best step?**

The next best step for this patient is reassurance since the diagnosis of mosquito bites can be established clinically. If the patient's diagnosis remained unclear based on the patient's history and physical exam findings, better visualization of the lesions could be achieved with a dermatoscope. Dermoscopy may reveal a single central punctum in the reaction area, which would further confirm the diagnosis of mosquito bites.[6,7] Dermoscopy can also be helpful in ruling out other conditions that may be on the differential. If a stinging insect such as a honeybee is the cause for the bite reaction, sometimes a residual stinger can be identified within the skin lesion. Spider bites would reveal dual puncta, as opposed to a single punctum.[6] Brown recluse spider bites can cause central skin necrosis with ulceration, which can also be better visualized with dermoscopy.[1]

5. **What are the most appropriate diagnostic modalities (i.e., labs, biopsies, scrapings, histological findings)?**

Mosquito bites are primarily a clinical diagnosis based on the patient's history and physical exam findings.[1] If a thorough history reveals likely arthropod exposure with classical skin findings on exam, there is no need for bloodwork, biopsy, or skin scraping.

6. **What would you expect to find in the histopathologic analysis?**

While biopsies and skin scrapings are not necessary for mosquito bite reactions, if a biopsy were to be obtained, histologic findings would include a wedge-shaped lymphocytic infiltrate with accentuation in the perivascular areas, interstitial eosinophils, and pronounced dermal edema.[3,5]

In sensitized patients, bullous skin reactions may occur after mosquito bites. Histologic findings of bullous reactions may reveal intraepidermal vesicles separated by thin strands of epidermis and pronounced edema of the papillary dermis.[5]

7. **Discuss the epidemiology of this disease**.

   a. **Discuss the incidence and prevalence:**

   Since insect bites are extremely common and are often recognized by the general population, most cases are not brought to the attention of a physician.[1] Mosquito bites tend to occur seasonally (during warmer, more humid months) or in areas that are warm and humid year-round. Bites are much more frequent in areas near stagnant water, since mosquitoes depend on an aquatic environment to breed and complete their life cycle.[3,6]

   b. **Discuss the sociodemographics of individuals affected by this disease (i.e., age, gender, race, geographic location, other risk factors):**

   Mosquito bites occur in every age group; however, more severe local reactions to mosquito bites are more common in young children.[4,6,8] Several factors identified as mosquito attractants include blood type, metabolic rate, body temperature, dark-colored clothing, the presence of lactic acid or ketones in sweat, and estrogens. In addition, drinking alcohol may attract mosquitoes, and eating bananas may attract certain types of *Anopheles* mosquitoes.[4,6] Individuals living in temperate climates are at increased risk for mosquito bites.[3,6]

8. Discuss the pathogenesis of this disease.

The pathogenesis of mosquito bites involves mechanical injury to the skin caused by the mosquito's mouthparts, which create a small puncture wound at the bite site in order to obtain blood from capillaries or small veins.[6] Local cutaneous reactions are a normal host immune response to the saliva injected by the mosquito when it bites.[6,8] The immediate cutaneous reaction involves the formation of a wheal with surrounding flare due to the release of histamine, serotonin, formic acid, or kinins.[1,3,6,8] IgE, IgG, and lymphocytes all play a role in local reactions to mosquito bites.[8] In atopic individuals and those who are sensitized to the specific biting mosquito, there may be a delayed local hypersensitivity reaction in response to the antigenic proteins in the mosquito's saliva.[6,8] The amount of serum IgE and IgG specific to mosquito saliva directly correlates with the size and severity of the delayed cutaneous reaction.[8]

9. What is the clinical presentation of this disease (i.e., grade, stage, subtypes)?

Clinical features of mosquito bite sites commonly include localized erythema and swelling that can begin as soon as 20 minutes after the bite has occurred.[6,8] These lesions usually measure 2–8 mm and occur in exposed areas of the body.[3] At 24–36 hours, pruritic papules may develop that take approximately 7–10 days to resolve.[8] Excoriations may also be present.[3]

"Skeeter syndrome," or large local reactions, may develop in younger children and atopic patients.[6–8] These reactions can begin within a few hours of the bite and present as large (2–10 cm or more), indurated areas of erythema, warmth, pain, pruritus, and swelling; they are sometimes accompanied with fever and fatigue.[6,8] This reaction is thought to be an immunologic response to allergens in the saliva of the biting mosquito.[7] Longer-lasting lesions can persist for weeks to months and can even reactivate when new bites occur in other areas of the body. Chronic and/or resolving lesions can develop hyperpigmentation, especially in patients with skin of color; this hyperpigmentation may last for several months.[3]

Systemic allergic reactions are rare but can occur in response to mosquito bites. Generalized urticaria and, even more rarely, signs of anaphylaxis can develop within minutes of being bitten. Patients who develop severe, recurrent anaphylaxis in response to mosquito bites are often eventually diagnosed with systemic mastocytosis.[6,8]

Atypical presentations involving exaggerated local bite reactions include the formation of large vesicles, nodules, tense bullae, and skin necrosis. While these reactions are uncommon, they may be a cardinal sign of an underlying hematologic malignancy (particularly chronic lymphocytic leukemia and, less commonly, mantle cell lymphoma). These findings can precede the diagnosis of malignancy; therefore, patients presenting with such exaggerated reactions to mosquito bites may warrant further investigation and screening.[3,5,6] In addition, Asian or Hispanic children and adolescents with chronic Epstein-Barr virus infection, natural killer (NK)–cell leukemia, or lymphoma may have similar bullous or necrotic skin reactions to mosquito bites (considered a hypersensitivity to mosquito bites).[3,5]

10. **Discuss treatment options**.

Treatment is primarily focused on improving the patient's symptoms of pruritus and erythema. Topical application of camphor or menthol lotion or gel can improve the itching sensation, and topical cooling with cold compresses or calamine lotion can reduce erythema and swelling.[3,6] Oral antihistamines are effective for reducing pruritus, erythema, and edema of the lesions, especially if large local reactions are present.[1,6] If the patient is very uncomfortable and experiencing burning, particularly over areas of excoriation, a topical anesthetic can be applied as well. Anesthetics containing pramoxine are widely available and have a low risk for contact dermatitis.[3]

For persistent pruritus or large local reactions, a topical corticosteroid (clobetasol 0.05% cream BID or mometasone 0.1% cream BID) can be used for a limited duration (2 weeks, or less if symptoms resolve).[1] Intralesional triamcinolone (10 mg/ml) can also be considered.[3,8] For severe, large local reactions (those that interfere with vision, eating/drinking, or movement) or systemic reactions, a short course of oral corticosteroids is recommended (prednisone 1 mg/kg to a maximum of 50 mg once daily for up to 1 week).[6,8]

In cases of superimposed infection, antibiotics can be given. Secondary infection is typically caused by staphylococci or, less commonly, streptococci.[3]

Rarely, in highly atopic, sensitized patients, anaphylaxis can occur (although more common with stinging insects).[1,3] In these cases, administration of intramuscular epinephrine at the first sign of anaphylaxis is imperative, and patients should carry an injectable epinephrine pen with them when doing any future outdoor activities.[1,6]

11. **Other important questions/details:**

Preventive measures

There are several measures one can take to prevent mosquito bites (Table 6.2). Simple behavioral modifications—along with the use of repellants, permethrin pretreated clothing, or a combination of techniques—can be used depending on the location and concentration of mosquitoes.[6,7,9]

Repellants are the mainstay of prevention and the most effective measure against mosquito bites.[6,7,9] Repellants typically function by either agonizing the olfactory receptors of arthropods, blocking their ability to recognize the scent of their prey, or by antagonizing receptors, converting an attracting scent to one that deters.[9] DEET (N,N-diethyl-3-methylbenzamide), picaridin, and lemon eucalyptus oil are the most widely used repellants; of these, DEET is the most effective, longest-acting, and provides the greatest coverage against a broad spectrum of arthropods.[7,9]

Permethrin, a compound that causes nervous system toxicity to insects that come in contact with it, can be used to treat clothing. The combined use of permethrin pretreated clothing and DEET repellant on exposed skin is one of the most efficacious regimens in preventing mosquito bites; this is the recommended prevention strategy in regions where mosquito-transmitted diseases are endemic.[9]

Table 6.2 Preventive Measures for Mosquito Bites[6,7,9]

PREVENTION TECHNIQUES	EXAMPLES	NOTES/DISCUSSION
Behavioral modifications	• Wearing protective, light-colored clothing • Limiting time outdoors after dusk • Limiting time near standing pools of water or marshes[7]	
Repellants	• DEET	• DEET repellants commonly come in 30–35% concentrations (lower concentrations are also available with a shorter duration of efficacy). • Sweating, swimming, washing, and being outside during rainfall can remove DEET and shorten protection time.[9] • Combination sunscreen/DEET repellant products are not recommended. Sunscreen should be applied first, followed by DEET, to maintain the efficacy of each. • DEET is considered safe in children 2 months or older.[7,9]
	• Picaridin	• Picaridin repellants are available in 7–20% concentrations; 20% is equally as effective as DEET (although for a shorter duration).[9] • Picaridin is odorless and nongreasy, unlike DEET.[7,9] • Picaridin is not considered safe in children less than 2 years of age.[7,9]
	• Lemon eucalyptus oil	• Lemon eucalyptus oil is a popular alternative to DEET and picaridin because it is a natural, plant-derived product.[7] • The lemon eucalyptus plant contains the active ingredient PMD (p-menthane-3,8-diol).[6,7,9] • PMD is about half as effective as DEET. • Safety in children below age 3 has not been established.[9]
Pretreated clothing	• Permethrin pretreated clothing	• Permethrin is applied to clothing and bedding (on both sides) for 30–45 seconds and then left to dry. • It remains effective for 2 weeks, even after several rounds of washing and drying.[9]
Other	• Mosquito netting • Window screens	• Mosquito netting and window screens are commonly used in areas with endemic mosquito-transmitted infections.[6]

Infectious diseases associated with mosquito bites

Many infectious diseases are transmitted by mosquitoes (Table 6.3). These diseases are region-specific and are spread by specific genera of mosquitoes; therefore, travelers may wish to take additional precautions—such as chemoprophylaxis in malaria-endemic areas—when traveling to those regions.[9,10]

Table 6.3 Common Mosquito-Transmitted Infections and Associated Regions[4,7,10]

MOSQUITO GENUS	DISEASE	REGION
Culex	West Nile virus	Americas, Africa, Middle East, Europe
	Japanese encephalitis	Asia, India, Australia
	St. Louis encephalitis	North America
	Western equine encephalitis	Western United States, Canada
	Rift Valley fever	Africa, Middle East
Anopheles	Malaria	Africa, South Asia, Southeast Asia, Middle East, Central and South America
Aedes	Yellow fever	Africa, South America
	Dengue	Caribbean, South and Central America, Asia
	Chikungunya	Worldwide
	Eastern equine encephalitis	Eastern United States, Caribbean
	Western equine encephalitis	Western United States, Canada
	Zika	Africa, Americas, Asia, Pacific

References

1. Marks JG, Miller JJ. *Lookingbill and Marks' Principles of Dermatology*. 6th ed. Philadelphia: Elsevier; 2018.
2. Wolff K, Johnson RA, Saavedra AP, Roh EK. *Fitzpatrick's Color Atlas and Synopsis of Clinical Dermatology*. 8th ed. New York: McGraw-Hill Education; 2017.
3. Bolognia JL, Jorizzo JL, Schaffer JV. *Dermatology*. Vol 2, 3d ed. Philadelphia: Elsevier Saunders; 2012.
4. James WD, Berger TG, Elston DM. *Andrews' Diseases of the Skin Clinical Dermatology*. 11th ed. London: Saunders Elsevier; 2011.
5. Weedon D. *Weedon's Skin Pathology*. London: Churchill Livingstone Elsevier; 2010.
6. Goddard J, Stewart PH. Insect and other arthropod bites. In: Post TW, ed. *UpToDate*. Waltham, MA: UpToDate; 2020. Accessed March 1, 2021. Available from: www.uptodate.com/contents/insect-and-other-arthropod-bites.
7. Juckett G. Arthropod bites. *Am Fam Physician*. December, 15, 2013;88(12):841–847. PMID: 24364549.
8. Kelso JM. Allergic reactions to mosquito bites. In: Post TW, ed. *UpToDate*. Waltham, MA: UpToDate; 2019. Accessed March 1, 2021. Available from: www.uptodate.com/contents/allergic-reactions-to-mosquito-bites.
9. Breisch NL. Prevention of arthropod and insect bites: Repellants and other measures. In: Post TW, ed. *UpToDate*. Waltham, MA: UpToDate; 2020. Accessed March 1, 2021. Available from: www.uptodate.com/contents/prevention-of-arthropod-and-insect-bites-repellants-and-other-measures.
10. Engleberg NC, DiRita VJ, Dermody TS. *Schaechter's Mechanisms of Microbial Disease*. 5th ed. Philadelphia: Lippincott Williams & Wilkins; 2012.

7

Hypopigmented, Coalescing, Oval-Shaped Macules with Fine Scaling

JOSIAH WILLIAMS AND CRISTIAN C. RIVIS

A 34-year-old male with no significant past medical history presents to clinic in August for evaluation of scaly lesions on his chest, upper back, and upper arms (Figure 7.1). He noticed the lesions when he returned from a beach trip 1 week ago. The patient has multiple 3- to 5-mm, well-circumscribed, hypopigmented, round and oval-shaped macules, some of which are overlapping and coalesce to form larger patches. They are mildly scaly and paler than the surrounding tan skin. They are not itchy, but they are distressing to the patient because of their appearance.

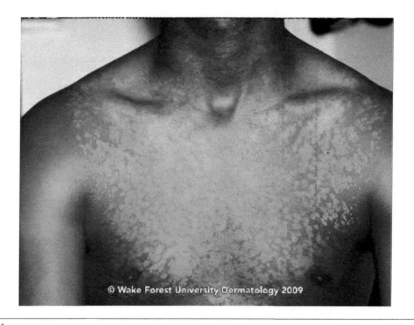

© Wake Forest University Dermatology 2009

Figure 7.1

1. **How would you describe the lesions?**
   Multiple hypopigmented, 3- to 5-mm, well-circumscribed, round and oval-shaped macules with a fine scale, some of which are coalescing into larger patches.

 DOI: 10.1201/9781003437987-7

2. What are the differential diagnoses (Table 7.1)?

Table 7.1   Differential Diagnoses for Hypopigmented, Coalescing, Oval-Shaped Macules with Fine Scaling

DIAGNOSIS	COMMENTS
Pityriasis versicolor (tinea versicolor)	Pityriasis versicolor typically presents as multiple 3- to 5-mm, well-circumscribed, round and oval-shaped, hypopigmented or hyperpigmented macules that may be white, reddish-brown, light pink, or tan.[1] They may exhibit a fine scale and are typically asymptomatic, though they may also present with mild pruritus.[2] Over time, they typically enlarge and coalesce to form irregularly shaped patches.[1]
Vitiligo	Vitiligo is an acquired disorder of depigmentation that results from selective destruction of melanocytes which causes white, non-scaling macules with distinct margins.[3]
Pityriasis alba	Pityriasis alba is a common hypopigmentation disorder most prevalent in children with a history of atopy. The lesions usually are initially faintly erythematous but develop into ill-defined, hypopigmented macules, patches, and sometimes plaques. They are often mildly scaly and pruritic.[4]
Mycosis fungoides	Mycosis fungoides is the most common form of cutaneous T-cell lymphoma and has a variable presentation. The hypopigmented variant presents with hypopigmented patches with a round or irregular border. Lesions may be pruritic and have an erythematous background.[5]
Seborrheic dermatitis	Seborrheic dermatitis typically presents as erythematous, scaly, pruritic lesions on the scalp, face, ears, chest, back, axillae, and/or groin.[6]
Pityriasis rosea	Pityriasis rosea is a common skin condition that is characterized by a single "herald patch" followed within a few weeks by multiple smaller patches and macules on the back, abdomen, chest, arms, and thighs.[7] The herald patch is typically 2–10 cm in size and is pink- to salmon-colored with fine central scale ("collarette"), while the subsequent lesions are smaller and violet or red-brown.[8] In darker Fitzpatrick skin phototypes, lesions may appear yellow to yellow-orange.[9]
Discoid lupus erythematosus	Skin lesions of classic discoid lupus erythematosus are typically indurated, well-circumscribed, scaly macules or papules with a violaceous color that gradually expand into coin-shaped patches and plaques.[10]

3. What is the most likely diagnosis?

The most likely diagnosis for this patient is pityriasis versicolor (tinea versicolor).

4. What is the best next step?

The best next step in a patient with suspected pityriasis versicolor is usually further evaluation with microscopy. A simple potassium hydroxide (KOH) direct mount of skin scrapings is the preferred method of visualizing the causal organisms, which are *Malassezia* subspecies. While many cases of pityriasis versicolor may be diagnosed clinically, microscopy confirms the diagnosis and can help differentiate pityriasis versicolor from other pathologies. A Wood's light can also be used to aid in diagnosis, though it is positive in less than 50% of cases.[2]

5. What are the most appropriate diagnostic modalities (i.e., labs, biopsies, scrapings, histological findings)

A KOH direct mount of skin scrapings is the preferred diagnostic test.[2] *Malassezia* species are yeasts with monopolar budding, and the mycelial form is responsible for pityriasis versicolor.[1,2] The appearance on the KOH direct mount classically looks like "spaghetti and meatballs," where the spherical bidding yeasts look like "meatballs" and the multibranching hyphae look like "spaghetti" noodles.[2]

6. **What would you expect to find in the histopathologic analysis?**

    Expected histopathologic findings of pityriasis versicolor include hyperkeratosis and acanthosis as well as a mild, superficial, perivascular infiltrate in the dermis. The *Malassezia* organisms should be visible on skin biopsy and display a similar "spaghetti and meatballs" appearance as seen on KOH direct mount, although stains such as periodic acid–Schiff may improve visualization.[11] In addition, a skin biopsy may look completely normal and is in the differential of normal histopathology. However, a skin biopsy is not required to confirm the diagnosis of pityriasis versicolor and is rarely performed.

7. **Discuss the epidemiology of this disease.**
    a. **Incidence and prevalence**

       Pityriasis versicolor is a common skin condition. It is particularly prevalent in summer months and in hot and humid climates due to its preference for warm and moist environments and its association with increased sebum production.[1,11,12] Prevalence is as high as 50% in some tropical countries and closer to 1% in cold climates, and pityriasis versicolor is responsible for up to 3% of dermatology office visits in temperate climates during summer months.[2,11] Lighter-skinned individuals are more likely to tan during the summer, which makes the hypopigmented lesions of pityriasis versicolor more visible[13]; this may contribute to the increased prevalence during warmer months.

    b. **Sociodemographics**

       Although it can occur at any age, pityriasis versicolor is most prevalent in adolescents and young adults.[13] Women and men are affected equally, and there is no ethnic predominance.[11,13]

8. **Discuss the pathogenesis of this disease.**

    Pityriasis versicolor is caused by *Malassezia* species, including *Malassezia furfur* and *Malassezia globosa*, which are normal skin flora. These organisms are dimorphic and typically live on the skin in yeast form. Once converted into their mycelial form, they spread into the superficial epidermis and cause the characteristic lesions of pityriasis versicolor.[1] A key factor that contributes to conversion from the yeast form to the mycelial form is increased sebaceous gland activity; therefore, hot and humid weather—as well as hyperhidrosis—can lead to pityriasis versicolor.[14] Dicarboxylic acids such as azelaic acid, which are breakdown products from *Malassezia* lipid metabolism, cause melanocyte damage. This melanocyte damage results in hypopigmented lesions. An inflammatory reaction to *Malassezia* causes the hyperpigmented lesions, and more organisms are present on these lesions compared with hypopigmented lesions.[15]

9. **What is the clinical presentation of this disease (i.e., grade, stage, subtypes)?**

Pityriasis versicolor most commonly presents as asymptomatic, hypo- and/or hyperpigmented macules and patches located on the upper arms, chest, back, and sometimes the face (Table 7.2).[1] Facial involvement is more common in children, while lesions on the trunk are more common in adolescents and young adults.[13] The lesions typically present as 3- to 5-mm, clearly demarcated, oval or round macules with a fine scale; over time, they may coalesce into larger patches of variable shape. Lesions vary in color and may be pale yellow, yellow-brown, dark brown, light brown, and sometimes reddish or pinkish. Patients usually present for cosmetic concerns, although mild pruritus may be present.[2]

Table 7.2 Clinical Variants of Pityriasis Versicolor

VARIANT FORM OF PITYRIASIS VERSICOLOR	CLINICAL PRESENTATION
Atrophying	Atrophying pityriasis versicolor typically presents as numerous hypopigmented or erythematous, depressed lesions varying in size from a few millimeters to several centimeters. They exhibit discrete desquamation and tend to be localized on the back and shoulders. Lesions are often uniform on the same patient.[16] The cause of atrophy is thought to be due to a delayed-type hypersensitivity reaction to *Malassezia* antigens.[17]
Hyperkeratotic	Hyperkeratotic patches on the face, forehead, cheeks, and scalp colonized with *Malassezia* species may be an atypical presentation of pityriasis versicolor.[18]
Recurrent and disseminated	Recurrent and disseminated pityriasis versicolor has been proposed as a separate entity from classic pityriasis versicolor. This variant is highly resistant to treatment and is associated with *Malassezia japonica*, a species not previously isolated in classic pityriasis versicolor.[19]

10. **Discuss treatment options.**

Although many treatment options are available for pityriasis versicolor, there is no consensus on the comparative effectiveness of these options.[20] Topical medications are first-line therapy for pityriasis versicolor and may be subdivided into nonspecific antifungal agents, which function primarily by shedding the stratum corneum to prevent further invasion, and specific antifungal drugs, which are directly fungicidal or fungistatic. In general, topical sprays or shampoos are preferred over creams and ointments because they are easier to apply to widespread areas and are less oily. Oral medications are second-line therapy used in treatment-resistant, severe, or widespread cases (Table 7.3).[11]

Based on current data, treatment should last from 1 to 4 weeks. Clinical improvement is usually not evident until 3–4 weeks after treatment.[1,20] Hypopigmented macules and patches will regain pigmentation over time with exposure to sunlight.[1]

Table 7.3   Common Treatments for Pityriasis Versicolor

MECHANISM	MEDICATION	USE
Nonspecific antifungals (primarily promote shedding of stratum corneum)	Zinc-pyrithione shampoo, selenium sulfide 2.5% shampoo, sulfur plus salicylic acid shampoo[11]	Apply for 5–10 minutes then wash off. Repeat daily for 7 days to 4 weeks.[1,20]
Fungistatic topical therapies	Ketoconazole 2% shampoo	Apply for 5 minutes then wash off. Repeat daily for 7 days.
	Ketoconazole 2% cream	Apply twice daily for 15 days.
	Clotrimazole 1%, econazole 1%, isoconazole 1%, miconazole 2% (available as shampoo or cream)	Shampoo: Apply for 5 minutes then wash off. Repeat daily for 7 days. Cream: Apply twice daily for 15 days.
Fungicidal topical therapies	Ciclopirox olamine 1%, terbinafine 1%[11] (available as shampoo or cream)	Shampoo: Apply for 5 minutes then wash off. Repeat daily for 7 days. Cream: Apply twice daily for 15 days.
Oral agents	Oral fluconazole 150 mg tablets[11]	Take 1–2 per week for 1–4 weeks.
	Oral itraconazole 200 mg tablets[11]	Take 1 daily for 7 days.

11. **Other important questions or details:**
    Dermatophyte infections

    Although pityriasis versicolor is also called tinea versicolor, it is not caused by dermatophyte species like other tinea infections. Dermatophyte infections, such as tinea corporis and tinea capitis, are mainly caused by *Microsporum*, *Epidermophyton*, and *Trichophyton* species. "Tinea" is Latin for "worm," and dermatophyte infections are typically named "tinea" followed by a descriptor of location (such as "capitis" for "head").[1] Despite the similar name, tinea versicolor should not be confused with dermatophyte infections.

    Seborrheic dermatitis

    Malassezia species play a role in the pathogenesis of both seborrheic dermatitis and pityriasis versicolor.[21] While pityriasis versicolor results from *Malassezia* yeasts converting to their mycelial form, seborrheic dermatitis is likely due to an inflammatory response to *Malassezia* species.[1,6]

References

1. Prawer S, Prawer S, Bershow A. Superficial fungal infections. In: Soutor C, Hordinsky MK, eds. *Clinical Dermatology*. New York, NY: McGraw-Hill Education; 2017.
2. Schwartz RA. Superficial fungal infections. *Lancet*. September 25–October 1, 2004; 364(9440):1173–1182.
3. Ezzedine K, Eleftheriadou V, Whitton M, van Geel N. Vitiligo. *Lancet*. July 4, 2015; 386(9988):74–84.
4. Givler DN, Basit H, Givler A. *Pityriasis Alba. StatPearls*. Treasure Island, FL: StatPearls Publishing LLC.; 2020.
5. Hodak E, Amitay-Laish I. Mycosis fungoides: A great imitator. *Clin Dermatol*. May–June, 2019;37(3):255–267.
6. Clark GW, Pope SM, Jaboori KA. Diagnosis and treatment of seborrheic dermatitis. *Am Fam Physician*. February 1, 2015;91(3):185–190.

7. Schadt C. Pityriasis Rosea. *JAMA Dermatol*. December 1, 2018;154(12):1496.
8. Zlotoff B, Keck LE, Padilla RS. Psoriasis and other papulosquamous diseases. In: Soutor C, Hordinsky MK, eds. *Clinical Dermatology*. New York: McGraw-Hill Education; 2017.
9. Jindal R, Chauhan P, Sethi S. Dermoscopic characterization of guttate psoriasis, pityriasis rosea, and pityriasis lichenoides chronica in dark skin phototypes: An observational study. *Dermatol Ther*. January, 2021;34(1):e14631.
10. Walling HW, Sontheimer RD. Cutaneous lupus erythematosus: Issues in diagnosis and treatment. *Am J Clin Dermatol*. 2009;10(6):365–381.
11. Karray M, McKinney WP. *Tinea (Pityriasis) Versicolor*. Treasure Island, FL: StatPearls; 2020.
12. Cunliffe WJ, Burton JL, Shuster S. The effect of local temperature variations on the sebum excretion rate. *Br J Dermatol*. December, 1970;83(6):650–654.
13. Kelly BP. Superficial fungal infections. *Pediatr Rev*. April, 2012;33(4):e22–e37.
14. Gupta AK, Batra R, Bluhm R, Faergemann J. Pityriasis versicolor. *Dermatol Clin*. July, 2003;21(3):413–429, v–vi.
15. Galadari I, el Komy M, Mousa A, Hashimoto K, Mehregan AH. Tinea versicolor: Histologic and ultrastructural investigation of pigmentary changes. *Int J Dermatol*. April, 1992;31(4):253–256.
16. Allegue F, Fachal C, Gonzalez-Vilas D, Zulaica A. Atrophying Pityriasis Versicolor. *Actas Dermosifiliogr*. June, 2018;109(5):455–457.
17. Yang YS, Shin MK, Haw CR. Atrophying pityriasis versicolor: Is this a new variant of pityriasis versicolor? *Ann Dermatol*. November, 2010;22(4):456–459.
18. Boralevi F, Marco-Bonnet J, Lepreux S, Buzenet C, Couprie B, Taïeb A. Hyperkeratotic Head and Neck *Malassezia* Dermatosis. *Dermatol*. 2006;212(1):36–40.
19. Romero-Sandoval K, Costa AA, Teixeira Sousa MG, et al. Recurrent and disseminated pityriasis versicolor: A novel clinical form consequent to Malassezia-host interaction? *Med Hypotheses*. November, 2017;109:139–144.
20. Hu SW, Bigby M. Pityriasis versicolor: A systematic review of interventions. *Archiv Dermatol*. 2010;146(10):1132–1140.
21. Faergemann J. Management of seborrheic dermatitis and pityriasis versicolor. *Am J Clin Dermatol*. March–April, 2000;1(2):75–80.

8

SCALY ANNULAR LESIONS

JESSIKA SANZ AND ADITI CHOKSHI

A 35-year-old white male with a history of diabetes and HIV presents to the clinic with an itchy rash on his right arm that started 4 months ago over the summer (Figure 8.1). The patient states that the itching is severe and that he has tried to treat it with topical emollients and hydrocortisone cream with no improvement. His current medications include emtricitabine, tenofovir, raltegravir, insulin glargine, and insulin lispro. The patient works in construction. Examination reveals an annular plaque with erythema and scaling.

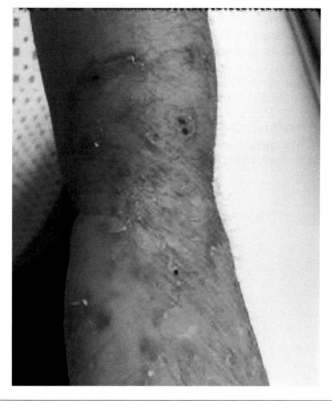

Figure 8.1   Physical exam findings.

1. How would you describe the lesion?

The arm has multiple asymmetric annular plaques measuring approximately 6 cm by 12 cm. The lesions have a central clearing and vesicles scattered over

          DOI: 10.1201/9781003437987-8

the plaques. The border is erythematous and advancing with sharply demarcated edges and peripheral scaling.

2. What are the differential diagnoses (Table 8.1)?

Table 8.1   Differential Diagnosis

DIAGNOSIS	COMMENTS
Tinea corporis	Tinea corporis is a dermatophyte infection that results in a superficial fungal infection affecting the face, trunk, and extremities. The lesions typically present as a circular, well-demarcated, scaly patch or plaque with a raised leading edge and central clearing. Lesions can present with differing levels of inflammation.[1]
Nummular dermatitis	Nummular dermatitis presents as red to purple, small papules and vesicles that coalesce to form exudative circular patches and later become lichenified patches with a discoid shape. The lesions may appear on the trunk, hands, or feet, but are predominantly found on the extensor surfaces of the forearms and shins. The disease course is often chronic and recurrent. Nummular dermatitis appears as papules or vesicles without a central clearing.[2]
Pityriasis versicolor	Pityriasis versicolor can cause hypo- or hyperpigmentation and commonly affects the chest and back due to high concentrations of sebaceous glands in these areas. Hypopigmented patches are often noticed during the summer months due to tanning of the surrounding skin. Scale may be present, and pruritus may also occur. There is minimal or absent erythema.[3]
Granuloma annulare (GA)	GA is a cutaneous granulomatous disease due to a noninfectious etiology. Localized GA is the most common variant and presents as flesh-colored to erythematous papules in an annular configuration. The lesions are commonly found on the dorsal hands or feet and appear more often in women under the age of 30. Generalized GA is characterized by the presence of ten or more of these skin lesions or by widespread annular plaques; this variant tends to have a later age of onset and a more chronic course. Granuloma annulare lesions lack scale and rarely affect the trunk.[4]
Psoriasis	The most common form of psoriasis is plaque psoriasis (psoriasis vulgaris). Lesions are monomorphic, sharply demarcated, erythematous plaques covered by silvery lamellar scales. Plaques may be sparse or may affect the entire body surface. Psoriasis can affect any area of the skin, but the most commonly affected locations include extensor surfaces; the scalp; and periumbilical, perianal, and retro-auricular regions.[5]

GA: Granuloma annulare

3. What is the most likely diagnosis?

The most likely diagnosis in this patient is tinea corporis.

4. What is the next best step?

The next best step in the management of this lesion is to take skin scrapings for wet mount preparation with potassium hydroxide (KOH). Once the
diagnosis of tinea corporis is confirmed, appropriate treatment should be
initiated as soon as possible. Any widespread dermatophyte infection should
raise suspicion for an immunocompromised state such as infection with
HIV.[6]

5. **What are the most appropriate diagnostic modalities (i.e., labs, biopsies, scrapings, histological findings)?**

Tinea corporis may be diagnosed with many different tests. Dermoscopy is a useful non-invasive diagnostic tool. Visualization of involvement of vellus hair on dermoscopy is an indication for initiation of systemic therapy.[7] If necessary, the diagnosis may be confirmed by other diagnostic modalities (Table 8.2).

Table 8.2   Diagnostic Modalities for Tinea Corporis

DIAGNOSTIC MODALITIES	DETAILS
Potassium hydroxide (KOH) wet mount preparation	Diagnosis can be achieved via direct examination of lesions and analysis of skin scrapings from the active edge of the lesion using a KOH wet mount preparation.[8] Before microscopic analysis, 10–20% KOH solution is applied to nail, hair, or skin scrapings. Low-temperature heating along with KOH preparation dissolves keratin and helps facilitate visualization of the dermatophyte.[1]
Fungal culture	A fungal culture is the gold standard to diagnose dermatophytosis, but it takes time for a definitive diagnosis. It is necessary if the results of other tests are inconclusive or the infection is resistant to treatment.[9] Sabouraud dextrose agar is used as an isolation medium for fungal cultures, and it may take between 5 days and 4 weeks for the culture to reveal growth.[1]
Wood's lamp examination	Wood's lamp examination is of limited prevalence due to the utilization of ultraviolet light in which dermatophytes found in the United States do not fluoresce. However, it may be useful in diagnosing pityriasis versicolor, which fluoresces pale yellow to white, or tinea capitis, which is caused by *Microsporum* species and fluoresces blue-green.[8]
Skin/nail biopsy	Skin or nail biopsy may assist in development of a treatment plan when there is no response to previous treatments, KOH microscopy is negative in patients with dystrophic nails, or in cases of difficult diagnoses.[8]
Uniplex polymerase chain reaction (PCR)	The conventional laboratory tests for tinea corporis infections such as direct microscopic examination with 10% KOH and fungal culture may be rather slow. PCR can be used to quickly identify the pathogen and initiate treatment, while a culture is simultaneously performed to confirm the identity and viability of the organism. This method also helps detect drug resistance. The sensitivity and specificity of the test compared with cultures are 80.1% and 80.6%, respectively.[7]

6. **What would you expect to find in the histopathologic analysis?**

Diagnosis of tinea corporis is typically established via dermoscopy or KOH staining. However, analysis of skin biopsy samples with hematoxylin and eosin (H&E) stain reveals a pathognomonic sign of a predominance of neutrophils in the stratum corneum. Septate branching hyphae may also be seen using special fungal stains such as periodic acid–Schiff (PAS) or Gömöri methenamine silver (GMS) stains.[7]

7. **Discuss the epidemiology of this disease.**

   a. **Discuss the incidence and prevalence:**

   The lifetime risk of acquiring tinea corporis is approximately 10–20%.[9] Dermatophytes are most common in developing countries, particularly in tropical and subtropical areas such as India due to their high temperature and humid environment.[7]

b. **Discuss the sociodemographics of individuals affected by this disease (i.e., age, gender, race, geographic location, other risk factors):**

Dermatophytes thrive in warm and moist environments and can be transmitted by direct contact with skin, household pets, or fomites. Patients with risk factors such as diabetes mellitus, lymphomas, immunocompromised status, older age, and Cushing's syndrome are more likely to contract a dermatophyte infection. Modifiable risk factors include wearing tight clothing or shoes with poor aeration, sharing clothing or towels with an infected person, and participating in physical activities that involve skin-to-skin contact, such as wrestling.

Genetic defects in innate and adaptive immunity may also increase risk for tinea infections. Patients with caspase recruitment domain-containing protein 9 (CARD9) deficiency are susceptible to dermatophyte dissemination to the lymph nodes,[7] and patients with low beta-defensin 4 are predisposed to all dermatophyte infections.[10]

8. **Discuss the pathogenesis of this disease**.

The term "tinea" refers to a disease caused by a fungal infection. A dermatophyte is the fungal organism that causes tinea.[11] Because dermatophytes utilize keratin to grow, infections are limited to hair, nails, and superficial skin.[8] Patients with tinea corporis are at risk of developing dermatophyte infections in other parts of the body due to autoinoculation.

Pathogenesis involves an intricate interaction between the host, agent, and environment.[7] The dermatophyte inoculates into the host's skin and adheres to keratinocytes.[6] Proteases, serine-subtilisins, and fungolysin mediate the process of penetration by digesting keratin into oligopeptides, which then act as immunogenic stimuli.[7]

In chronic dermatophytosis, mannans—fungal cell wall glycoproteins that inhibit lymphocytes—are produced by *Trichophyton rubrum*. Decreased function of T helper 17 (Th17) cells leads to impaired production of interleukin 17 (IL-17) and interleukin-22 (IL-22), cytokines that function to clear fungal infections, resulting in chronic dermatophyte infection.[7]

9. **What is the clinical presentation of this disease (i.e., grade, stage, subtypes)?**

Dermatophyte infections can be classified into multiple clinical subtypes (Table 8.3).

Prepubertal children are more likely to develop tinea corporis and tinea capitis, whereas adolescents and adults are more prone to develop tinea cruris, tinea pedis, and tinea unguium.[11]

Table 8.3 Clinical Subtypes of Dermatophyte Infections

CLINICAL SUBTYPE	CHARACTERISTICS
Tinea corporis (ringworm)	• Includes tinea gladiatorum and tinea faciei. • Appears as single or numerous annular lesions with central clearing; raised, erythematous edge; peripheral scale; and sharp margination on the torso, extremities, or face. • Topical corticosteroids usage can result in absence of typical elevated edges and the central clearing typically seen in lesions.[8]
Tinea capitis	• Dermatophyte infection of the scalp. • The most common dermatophytosis in children. • Infection is commonly caused by improper hygiene, overcrowding, and fomites. • Well-demarcated alopecia and scarring occur during infection.[8] • Some evidence that antifungal resistance may not be common in tinea capitis.[7]
Tinea cruris	• Dermatophyte infection of the groin, also known as jock itch. • The prevalence is higher in men compared to women. More common in hot and humid environments. • Thrives in moist environments such as occlusive clothing or tight footwear. • Most commonly involves the proximal medial thighs with extension to the buttocks and abdomen. However, the scrotum is spared. • Examination of the feet should be performed to evaluate for a possible source of infection.[8]
Tinea pedis	• Dermatophyte infection of the foot, also known as athlete's foot. • The interdigital form is the most prevalent subtype and is characterized by fissuring, softening, and scaling of skin in the interdigital spaces of the fourth and fifth toes that cause pruritus and burning. • *Trichophyton rubrum* infection causes a moccasin-like distribution pattern in which the plantar skin develops chronic scale and becomes hyperkeratotic. • Vesiculobullous form of tinea pedis develops on the soles of the feet with vesicles, pustules, and bullae.[8]
Tinea unguium (onychomycosis)	• Dermatophyte infection of the nail. • Risk factors include aging, diabetes, tight shoes, and pre-existing tinea pedis infection. • Diagnosis should be confirmed via histologic analysis of the nail specimen with periodic acid–Schiff (PAS) staining before treatment is initiated because onychomycosis requires prolonged therapy and may be expensive. Less sensitive diagnostic methods such as KOH microscopy or fungal cultures can be used if the PAS stain is unavailable.[8]
Tinea barbae	• Most commonly affects the skin and hair follicles of the beard and mustache area. • Occurs most often in males, hirsute females, and farmworkers. • May cause scaling, follicular pustules, and erythema.[8]
Tinea manuum	• Dermatophyte infection of one or both hands. • Often occurs in patients with pre-existing tinea pedis infection. • The palmar surface is dry and thickened. Involvement of the fingernails may result in vesicles and minimal scaling.[8]

10. **Discuss treatment options.**

Tinea corporis generally responds to topical agents such as terbinafine cream. However, in patients with substantial diseases, immunocompromised patients, or failure with topical treatment, oral antifungal agents may be used (Table 8.4).[11] Utilization of topical fungal allylamines is associated with higher cure rates and shorter treatment courses than in treatment with fungistatic azoles.[8]

Table 8.4 Treatment Options for Tinea Corporis

TREATMENT	DOSING	MECHANISM OF ACTION
Clotrimazole	• 1% cream, ointment, or solution applied twice daily for 2–3 weeks[1]	Binds to phospholipids and inhibits the biosynthesis of ergosterol and other sterols
Ketoconazole	• 2% cream, shampoo, gel, or foam applied once daily for 2–3 weeks[1]	necessary for fungal cell membrane production, therefore preventing the growth of the fungus.
Miconazole	• 2% cream, ointment, solution, lotion, or powder applied twice daily for 2–3 weeks[1]	
Naftifine	• 1% cream applied once daily • 1% or 2% gel applied twice daily for 2–3 weeks[1]	Inhibits the enzyme 2,3-epoxidase, thereby inhibiting the biosynthesis of ergosterol.
Terbinafine	• 1% cream, gel, or spray solution once or twice daily • 250 mg orally once daily for 2 weeks[1]	Inhibits the enzyme squalene monooxygenase, thereby inhibiting the biosynthesis of ergosterol.
Itraconazole	• 100 mg once daily for 2 weeks • 200 mg once daily for 1 week (give capsules with food)[1]	Binds to phospholipids and inhibits the biosynthesis of ergosterol and other sterols required for cell membrane production, therefore preventing the growth of the fungus.
Fluconazole	• 150–200 mg once weekly • 50–100 mg/day for 2–4 weeks[1]	Binds to phospholipids and inhibits the biosynthesis of ergosterol and other sterols required for cell membrane production, therefore preventing the growth of the fungus.
Griseofulvin	• 500–1000 mg once daily for 2–4 weeks[1]	Inhibits fungal cell mitosis and nuclear acid synthesis. Interferes with the function of cytoplasmic microtubules.

mg: milligrams

11. **Other important questions/details:**
    Complications

    Tinea corporis can cause severe itching, and scratching may cause skin abrasions that increase the risk for bacterial superinfection. After starting systemic fungal treatment, patients may experience dermatophytid reaction or auto-eczematization, a secondary dermatitic eruption. This is likely due to an immunologic reaction to fungal antigens. On rare occasions, patients may experience a psoriatic flare triggered by tinea infection. Individuals with tinea infections may also experience negative psychological, social, and occupational impacts.[9]

Special populations

Patients with significant renal and hepatic impairment should be cautious in taking certain antifungal medications. Terbinafine clearance is reduced in patients with renal impairment, and itraconazole should be avoided in patients with hepatic impairment. Terbinafine therapy falls under Food and Drug Administration (FDA) pregnancy category B; however, no accepted guidelines are available for treatment during pregnancy, and therapy should be individualized based on the risks and benefits. Patients with HIV may present with more widespread involvement, but classic characteristics may not appear due to suppressed immunity.[7]

Chronic dermatophytosis

Chronic dermatophytosis is characterized by identification of *T. rubrum* in microscopy and by the involvement of at least four body sites. Chronic infection may involve episodes of remission and exacerbation.[7]

References

1. Yee G, Al Aboud AM. Tinea corporis. In: *StatPearls*. Treasure Island, FL: StatPearls Publishing; August 8, 2022.
2. Martínez-Blanco J, García-González V, González-García J, Suárez-Castañón C. Dermatitis numular: Presentación de dos casos pediátricos [Nummular dermatitis: Report of two cases in children]. *Arch Argent Pediatr.* 2016;114(4):e241–e244. doi:10.5546/aap.2016.e241
3. Hudson A, Sturgeon A, Peiris A. Tinea Versicolor. *JAMA.* 2018;320(13):1396. doi:10.1001/jama.2018.12429
4. Keimig EL. Granuloma Annulare. *Dermatol Clin.* 2015;33(3):315–329. doi:10.1016/j.det.2015.03.001
5. Boehncke WH, Schön MP. Psoriasis. *Lancet.* 2015;386(9997):983–994. doi:10.1016/S0140-6736(14)61909-7
6. Rouzaud C, Hay R, Chosidow O, et al. Severe dermatophytosis and acquired or innate immunodeficiency: A review. *J Fungi (Basel).* December 31, 2015;2(1):4. doi:10.3390/jof2010004
7. Sahoo AK, Mahajan R. Management of tinea corporis, tinea cruris, and tinea pedis: A comprehensive review. *Indian Dermatol Online J.* 2016;7(2):77–86. doi:10.4103/2229-5178.178099
8. Hainer BL. Dermatophyte infections. *Am Fam Physician.* 2003;67(1):101–108.
9. Leung AK, Lam JM, Leong KF, Hon KL. Tinea corporis: An updated review. *Drugs Context.* 2020;9:2020–5-6. Published 2020 Jul 20. doi:10.7573/dic.2020–5-6
10. Jaradat SW, Cubillos S, Krieg N, et al. Low DEFB4 copy number and high systemic hBD-2 and IL-22 levels are associated with dermatophytosis. *J Invest Dermatol.* 2015;135(3):750–758. doi:10.1038/jid.2014.369
11. Ely JW, Rosenfeld S, Seabury Stone M. Diagnosis and management of tinea infections. *Am Fam Physician.* 2014;90(10):702–710.

9

RED AND TAN MACULES AND PATCHES

ISABELLA DREYFUSS AND CRISTIAN C. RIVIS

A 50-year-old female presents to the clinic for evaluation of asymmetric, poorly defined, hyperpigmented macules on her face and arms (Figure 9.1). The patient first noticed the lesions approximately 2 days ago after receiving laser treatment for hair removal. The patient has not attempted any treatments for the new lesions.

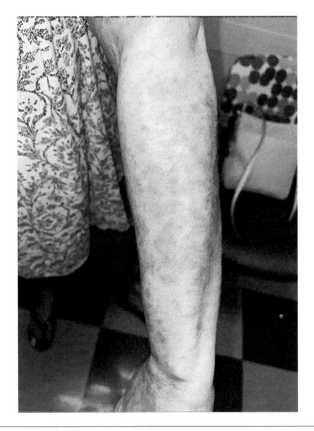

Figure 9.1 Patient presentation.

DOI: 10.1201/9781003437987-9

1. How would you describe the lesion?

The lesions range from approximately 2 to 5 mm in diameter and are red and tan, circular macules of hyperpigmentation along a similar distribution of where the patient had hair removed.[1]

2. What are the differential diagnoses (Table 9.1)?

Table 9.1   Differential Diagnosis for Red and Tan Macules and Patches

DIAGNOSIS	COMMENTS
Melasma	Melasma appears as dark brown, irregular macules on the sun-exposed areas of the face, cervical region, and neckline. Melasma has well-defined borders and will appear light brown on Wood's lamp examination.[2]
Solar lentigines	Solar lentigines are flattened, acquired pigmented lesions on sun-damaged skin ranging in size from 0.3 to 2 cm. Lesions range from yellow-tan to black and are often split by fine wrinkles. Lesions often slowly increase in number and size. Solar lentigines are common in the middle aged and elderly.[3]
Tinea versicolor	Tinea versicolor, or pityriasis versicolor, is a fungal infection caused by the fungi from the genus *Malassezia*. Tinea versicolor affects teens and young adults and results in small, discolored, oval patches on the skin. These patches often merge into larger, irregular patches that vary from yellow, to brown, to red, to pink. Tinea versicolor more commonly presents with hypopigmented lesions.[4,5]
Acanthosis nigricans	Acanthosis nigricans consists of poorly defined, coarse, velvety, brown-to-black regions of hyperpigmentation. It presents on the posterior and lateral folds of the neck, armpits, and navel, usually in diabetic or obese patients.[6] Patient-specific characteristics, such as a history of diabetes, can help distinguish between acanthosis nigricans from other conditions.
Lichen planus pigmentosus (LPP)	LPP is characterized by a photodistribution of irregularly shaped dyschromia on the forehead, temples, and neck. LPPs are oval-shaped, hyperpigmented, gray-blue or brown-black macules and/or patches.[7]
Macular amyloidosis	Macular amyloidosis is a chronic cutaneous amyloidosis with pruritic, hyperkeratotic, gray-brown macules on the trunk and extremities. These lesions have been seen in a rippled pattern on the upper back from macules that have coalesced.[8] Macular amyloidosis typically appears in a symmetrical pattern.[9]
Erythema dyschromicum perstans morphea (EDPM)	EDPM, also called ashy dermatosis, is a gray, well-defined, oval or irregular group of patches of dermal macular hyperpigmentation on the face, neck, and trunk. EDPM is a form of acquired dermal macular hyperpigmentation.[10] Lesions of EPDM progress from a reddish color to gray and have a pronounced border.[9]
Discoid lupus erythematosus (DLE)	DLE is a chronic skin condition of inflammation and scarring on the face, ears, scalp, and nasal labial folds, concurrent with lupus. Patients report mild pruritus, pain, and burning of the lesions and typically have systemic involvement within 3 years of diagnosis. Lesions of DLE are inflamed red patches that often crust.[11]
Post-inflammatory hyperpigmentation (PIH)	PIH is a condition characterized by increased melanin deposition within the skin following endogenous or exogenous injury. The deposition occurs within the dermal or epidermal layers of the affected skin, causing darker tan, brown, or bluish-gray discoloration depending on the original skin tone. Melanin deposition may result as a response to endogenous inflammatory insults such as psoriasis, acne vulgaris, or atopic dermatitis, or exogenous inflammation such as burns or irritant contact dermatitis. The distribution of hyperpigmentation corresponds to the sites of injury and is otherwise asymptomatic. While PIH can occur in all skin phenotypes, it is more prevalent in Fitzpatrick skin types IV, V, and VI. Clinical history is key to this diagnosis. A biopsy revealing increased dermal or epidermal melanin deposition can be helpful in the absence of a clear history.[12]

3. **What is the most likely diagnosis?**

The most likely diagnosis in this patient is post-inflammatory hyperpigmentation (PIH).

4. **What is the next best step?**

The next best step in the management of these multiple lesions with clinical suspicion for PIH is history and physical evaluation for acne and other risk factors. PIH is commonly a clinical diagnosis, although evaluation with Wood's lamp and occasionally biopsy may be used to aid in diagnosis.

5. **What are the most appropriate diagnostic modalities (i.e., labs, biopsies, scrapings, histological findings)?**

Further evaluation can be performed with dermoscopy and visualization of dermal melanosis with gray-purple-brown discoloration. Dermoscopy is a useful diagnostic tool for evaluation of PIH, with examination of five parameters including vessels, scales, follicular findings, other structures such as color and morphology, and clues such as pathological correlation.[13] Further tools for evaluation include Wood's lamp examination; this accentuates the lesion borders of epidermal PIH. PIH can be histologically classified through the pigmentation displayed on Wood's light examination of 320–400 nm.[14] Ultraviolet (UV) or black light Wood's lamp differentiates epidermal versus dermal hypermelanosis. Hypopigmented macules are also excluded under Wood's lamp.

Biopsy may provide definitive differential diagnosis if necessary. Standard hematoxylin-eosin stain and silver stain can locate the layer of involvement but are not commonly used for diagnosis.

6. **What would you expect to find in the histopathologic analysis?**

PIH has increased melanin in keratinocytes and dermal macrophages, a differentiating factor from melasma. Melanin deposits on the upper dermis form around blood vessels, which triggers inflammation. The darkening of the basal layer is thought to be from chronic histologic inflammation, reactive oxygen species, and cytokines.[2] Giant melanosomes are occasionally found within the epidermis. Melanocytes stimulate dendritic proliferation via tyrosinase, yet the exact pathogenesis of PIH is still not completely understood.[1]

7. **Discuss the epidemiology of this disease**.

a. **Discuss the incidence and prevalence:**

PIH is most common in patients with Fitzpatrick skin types III–VI. PIH is found to be more present in African Americans with acne and other skin conditions. Approximately 65.3% of African American, 52.7% of Hispanic, and 47.4% of Asian patients developed acne-induced PIH.[9]

b. **Discuss the sociodemographics of individuals affected by this disease (i.e., age, gender, race, geographic location, other risk factors):**

PIH occurs more commonly in people of color, such as African Americans, Hispanics, Asians, and Native Americans. PIH is most prevalent in the northeastern region of the United States and with adult patients in their twenties to forties.[1] Risk factors include an imbalance of hormone levels, as seen commonly in pregnancy, acne, and atopic dermatitis.

8. Discuss the pathogenesis of this disease.

PIH results from the overproduction of melanin, known as hypermelanosis, or abnormal deposition of melanin within the dermal layer. PIH often occurs after inflammation from acne, eczema, lichen planus, allergic reactions, or other insults resulting in cutaneous inflammation, such as surgery, microdermabrasion, or chemical peels.[9] Damaged basal keratinocytes release melanin that are phagocytosed by melanophages and cause a blue-grayish tint to patients.[11] Interactions between keratinocyte growth factor receptor and interleukin-1α induce melanin deposition; this receptor is increased in the context of the mesenchymal-epithelial interactions found in PIH. Leukotrienes (LT)-C4 and LT-D4 and reactive oxygen species nitric oxide may have melanocyte-stimulating properties contributing to disease pathogenesis.[9] The duration of PIH most often depends on the cutaneous depth and concentration of epidermal melanin; greater depth and higher concentrations of melanin are associated with longer PIH duration. Other factors that cause PIH include atopic dermatitis, allergic contact dermatitis, trauma, psoriasis, lichen planus, drug eruptions, and cosmetic procedures.

9. What is the clinical presentation of this disease (i.e., grade, stage, subtypes) (Table 9.2)?

Table 9.2   Classification of PIH

CLASSIFICATION	CHARACTERISTICS
Epidermal melanosis	• Histological examination reveals large amounts of melanin with regular amounts of melanocytes • Borders are sharply demarcated with dark brown coloring
Dermal melanosis	• Histological evaluation reveals melanin within the dermal layer between bundles of collagen within melanophages, with regular amounts of melanin in the epidermal layer • Borders are not sharply demarcated, but the lesions are brown-gray • Certain treatments, such as hydroquinone, are not as responsive to dermal melanosis because of melanin incontinence and phagocytosis of melanosomes
Mixed type	• Histological evaluation reveals an increase in melanin in the epidermis and melanophages within the dermis layer • Commonly caused by trauma and inflammation from acne • Bleaching therapy is only successful in the epidermal layer of this form of PIH

PIH: Post-inflammatory hyperpigmentation

10. Discuss treatment options.

Treatment for PIH includes hydroquinone, sunscreen, chemexfoliation, depigmentation agents, and laser or light therapy (Table 9.3). Photoprotection is considered a pre-therapy and/or means to prevent the creation and worsening of PIH.[6] Many patients often exacerbate their hyperpigmentation from acne with harmful UV radiation.

The standard course of therapy for PIH starts with a combination of hydroquinone and tretinoin. Chemical peels with glycolic acid and salicylic acid can also be effective. Patients with even darker lesions may benefit from laser therapy and fractional photothermolysis.[1] Clinicians should exercise judgment to balance the possible skin irritation and additional hyperpigmentation caused from laser therapy.

Table 9.3 Treatment Options for PIH

TREATMENT TYPE	TREATMENT	INDICATIONS	MECHANISM OF ACTION	NOTES
Topical tyrosinase inhibitors	Hydroquinone[8]	Photoaging lesions and exogenous ochronosis	Converts DOPA to melanin by inhibiting tyrosinase	• First-line therapy • Decreases lesion size • Use with retinoids to increase efficacy
	Azelaic acid[10]	Depigmenting skin from mild-to-moderate acne	Asserts selective cytotoxic effects on abnormal melanocytes	• Belongs to the class of dicarboxylic acids • Isolates pityriasis versicolor
	Arbutin	Epidermal hyperpigmentation	Inhibits melanosome maturation	• Commonly used in solar lentigines, melasma, and freckles
Chemexfoliation	Glycolic acid	Burns in African Americans with Fitzpatrick skin types IV–VI and facial PIH	Increases dermal collagen synthesis, disperses basal layer melanin, and induces epidermolysis	• Naturally occurring α-hydroxy acid • Available in chemical peels
	Salicylic acid	Post-skin reaction to chemical peels, also used in Fitzpatrick skin types V and VI	Induces keratolysis, disrupts intercellular lipid epithelioid cells	• Beta-hydroxy treatment formed from willow tree bark
Laser/light therapy	Blue light photodynamic therapy	Sun-damaged skin	Kills targeted cells and activated by aminolevulinic acid	• Requires 3–14 days of recovery
	Fractional photothermolysis	Acne scars, surgical scars, photodamaged skin, and facial rhytides[15]	Ablates skin with laser treatment, reignites skin resurfacing	• Stratum corneum remains intact • Microtreatment zones of thermolysis at specific depths
	YAG laser	Fractional photothermolysis on darker skin needing intensely pulsed light[15,16]	Converts radiant optical energy into thermal energy at 1,064 nm or via blue light	• Longer wavelengths penetrate deeper with selective absorption • Uses dermal targets
Depigmentation agents	Tretinoin[8]	Ethnic patients desiring skin lightening	Modulates cell proliferation, differentiation, and apoptosis	• Leads to less irritation as an analogue of vitamin A

DOPA: dihydroxyphenylalanine, **PIH:** post-inflammatory hyperpigmentation; **YAG:** yttrium, aluminum, garnet

11. **Other important questions/details:**
    a. **Risk of treatment with PIH**

    Chemical peels are often used as a lightening procedure for PIH, yet great care should be taken to avoid papillary dermis penetration. Papillary dermis penetration from chemical peels can potentially result in dyspigmentation, keloid formation, and hypertrophic scarring. Cross-reactions with other oral and topical medications, herpes simplex virus infections, and scarring infections can also occur.[1] Common adverse effects of treatment of PIH with chemical peels include erythema, burning sensation, and vesiculation.

    b. **Hyperpigmentation may be caused by medications**

    Many oral contraceptives can cause hyperpigmentation, which can be mistaken for PIH. Drug-induced hyperpigmentation results from anti-malarials, amiodarone, chemotherapy drugs, and other heavy metals.

References

1. Ogbechie-Godec OA, Elbuluk N. Melasma: An up-to-date comprehensive review. *Dermatol Ther (Heidelb)*. 2017;7(3):305–318.
2. Cestari TF, Dantas LP, Boza JC. Acquired hyperpigmentations. *An Bras Dermatol*. 2014;89(1):11–25.
3. Bolognia J, Schaffer JV, Cerroni L. *Dermatology*. 4th ed.
4. Prawer S, Prawer S, Bershow A. Superficial fungal infections. In: Soutor C, Hordinsky MK, eds. *Clinical Dermatology*. 4th ed. New York, NY: McGraw-Hill Education; 2017.
5. Schwartz RA. Superficial fungal infections. *Lancet*. September 25–October 1, 2004; 364(9440):1173-1182.
6. Passeron T. Post-inflammatory hyperpigmentation. *Ann Dermatol Venereol*. 2016;143 (Suppl 2):S15–S19.
7. Leung N, Oliveira M, Selim MA, McKinley-Grant L, Lesesky E. Erythema dyschromicum perstans: A case report and systematic review of histologic presentation and treatment. *Int J Womens Dermatol*. 2018;4(4):216–222.
8. Shenoy A, Madan R. Post-inflammatory hyperpigmentation: A review of treatment strategies. *J Drugs Dermatol*. 2020;19(8):763–768.
9. Davis EC, Callender VD. Postinflammatory hyperpigmentation: A review of the epidemiology, clinical features, and treatment options in skin of color. *J Clin Aesthet Dermatol*. 2010;3(7):20–31.
10. Rossi AB, Leyden JJ, Pappert AS, et al. A pilot methodology study for the photographic assessment of post-inflammatory hyperpigmentation in patients treated with tretinoin. *J Eur Acad Dermatol Venereol*. 2011;25(4):398–402.
11. Techapichetvanich T, Wanitphakdeedecha R, Iamphonrat T, et al. The effects of recombinant human epidermal growth factor containing ointment on wound healing and post inflammatory hyperpigmentation prevention after fractional ablative skin resurfacing: A split-face randomized controlled study. *J Cosmet Dermatol*. 2018;17(5):756–761.
12. Kaufman BP, Aman T, Alexis AF. Postinflammatory hyperpigmentation: Epidemiology, clinical presentation, pathogenesis and treatment. *Am J Clin Dermatol*. 2018;19(4):489-503.
13. Errichetti E. Dermoscopy of inflammatory dermatoses (inflammoscopy): An up-to-date overview. *Dermatol Pract Concept*. 2019;9(3):169–180.

14. Nieuweboer-Krobotova L. Hyperpigmentation: Types, diagnostics and targeted treatment options. *J Eur Acad Dermatol Venereol.* 2013;27(Suppl 1):2–4.

15. Geronemus RG. Fractional photothermolysis: Current and future applications. *Lasers Surg Med.* 2006;38(3):169–176.

16. Sirithanabadeekul P, Srieakpanit R. Intradermal tranexamic acid injections to prevent post-inflammatory hyperpigmentation after solar lentigo removal with a Q-switched 532-nm Nd:YAG laser. *J Cosmet Laser Ther.* 2018;20(7–8):398–404.

10
PATCHES OF HAIR LOSS

ISABELLA DREYFUSS AND BROOKE W. SLIGH

A 36-year-old Caucasian male with a family history of male pattern baldness presents to the clinic for evaluation of hair loss on the back of his scalp (Figure 10.1). There are smooth, round, sharply demarcated patches of hair loss with exclamation point hairs on the periphery of the patches. The patient first noticed the hair loss approximately 1 year ago, but it has recently progressed to encompass entire areas of the scalp. Lately, he has been stressed due to an upcoming accounting exam. The patient has not attempted any treatments for the lesions.

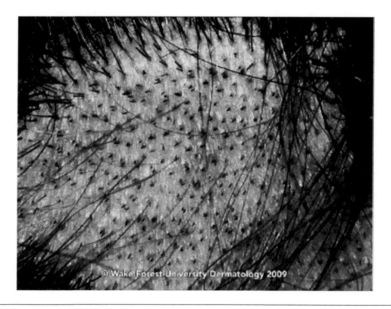

Figure 10.1 Patient presentation.

1. **How would you describe the lesion?**
   The lesions are randomly dispersed over the scalp and appear as well-defined regions of uniform hair loss, exposing the underlying epidermis. The lesions vary in size but are typically circular and nontender to palpation. Additionally, they are not erythematous, purulent, or pruritic.

                    DOI: 10.1201/9781003437987-10

2. What are the differential diagnoses (Table 10.1)?

Table 10.1   Differential Diagnoses for Patches of Hair Loss

DIAGNOSIS	COMMENTS
Trichotillomania	Trichotillomania is a psychological disorder in which patients have the impulse to pull their own hair out, resulting in irregular or tonsural patches of hair loss. The condition often presents in teenage girls. Physical exam would reveal broken hairs that are firmly attached to the scalp.[1]
Tinea capitis (TC)	TC is a fungal disease often found in children. It is associated with patchy hair loss, scalp inflammation and scaling, and pruritus.[2] Typically, TC is passed between children via pets or shared items such as hairbrushes, hats, and pillowcases.[3] Trichoscopy findings include comma hairs, which are misshapen due to the presence of fungi.[2,4]
Androgenetic alopecia	Androgenetic alopecia is a non-scarring, hereditary condition that differentially affects men and women. Men typically experience a regressing hairline and thinning on the peak of the head; women experience a widespread thinning with preservation of the hairline.[5] Clinically, androgenetic alopecia is insidious in nature.[6] In ambiguous presentations, a biopsy can differentiate this disease from others.[7]
Central centrifugal cicatricial alopecia (CCCA)	CCCA is a gradual, inflammatory, scarring alopecia that originates on the central region of the scalp and expands.[8,9] It is typically found in African American females and can be attributed to family history, genetics, and haircare (heat, damaging chemical relaxers, and tight hairstyles).[9,10] CCCA—previously known as hot comb alopecia or follicular degeneration syndrome—presents with pain, itching, and tingling.[9]
Telogen effluvium (TE)	TE is classically a non-scarring, widespread, acute alopecia marked by intense shedding of hair.[11] TE is precipitated by factors such as fever, infection, significant surgery, trauma, childbirth, heavy metal consumption, iron deficiency, excess dieting, vaccinations, and medications. Less commonly, TE can present as a chronic, slow-onset hair loss.[8,11]
Alopecia areata (AA)	AA is an autoimmune disorder that causes a non-scarring, patchy hair loss involving the scalp. Typically, the lesions are minor and circular; however, they can evolve to involve the entire scalp (alopecia totalis) or entire body (alopecia universalis).[8] The disease is most often asymptomatic, but it can rarely be pruritic, painful, or paresthetic.[12]

3. What is the most likely diagnosis?
The most likely diagnosis in this patient is alopecia areata (AA).

4. What is the next best step?
The next best step after history and physical examination is dermoscopy—specifically, trichoscopy.[6] Trichoscopy is the non-invasive, dermoscopic analysis of the hair and scalp.[2] After visualization of AA with trichoscopy, a hair pull test and biopsy can aid in diagnosing AA; however, a biopsy is not required to make the diagnosis.[6]

5. What are the most appropriate diagnostic modalities (i.e., labs, biopsies, scrapings, histological findings)?
AA is a clinical diagnosis made through a thorough history and physical exam using dermoscopy and a hair pull test.[6] In AA, dermoscopy will reveal yellow

dots (follicular cavities obstructed by oil and keratin),[13] black dots (splintered hair fragments),[2] broken hairs, exclamation point hairs, and short vellus hairs, distinguishing AA from other causes of hair loss.[8] A hair pull test, which involves securely pulling or tugging on a bundle of 50–60 hairs in multiple locations on the scalp, may also aid in diagnosis. In a positive hair pull test, 10% or more of the pulled hairs will fall out. A positive hair pull test signifies ongoing hair sloughing, which is present in AA, numerous scarring alopecias, and telogen effluvium.[10]

Although a skin biopsy is not typically required, it may help discern AA from other conditions, such as early scarring alopecia.[8]

6. **What would you expect to find in the histopathologic analysis?**

While analyzing both transverse and horizontal histopathological segments for precision, hair follicles suffering from AA will exhibit an inflammatory infiltrate—specifically, eosinophils and CD4+ and CD8+ T-cells—encompassing the bulbs in the anagen, or growing, phase.[8] Some studies have compared this histopathology to a "swarm of bees" given the various cell types.[12,14] Further evaluation may reveal edema, apoptosis, macrophages, and foreign body giant cells surrounding the hair bulb.[14]

The histological features and various stages of a single hair follicle help distinguish acute and chronic patches of AA.[15] Normally, a hair follicle proceeds from the anagen to the catagen to the telogen phase, where it can re-enter the anagen phase and continue to grow. However, in an early patch of AA, the follicles undergo a quick transition from the anagen phase to a disorderly catagen and telogen phase.[8] Chronic patches consist of large numbers of catagen- and telogen-phase follicles, miniature hairs, and many hair follicles lacking terminal hair filaments. Additionally, in chronic patches of AA, pigmentary incontinence—a collection of melanin granules—can be seen in the dermal papilla of hair bulbs.[8,14] Finally, in the resolution phase, inflammation subsides, and the quantity of terminal anagen hairs expands due to extension and development of miniature hairs.[15]

7. **Discuss the epidemiology of this disease**.

   a. **Discuss the incidence and prevalence:**

   The prevalence of AA worldwide is about 1 in 1,000 people, and the lifetime likelihood is about 2%.[6] There is an association between AA and other immune diseases including type 1 diabetes mellitus, systemic lupus erythematosus, thyroid conditions, vitiligo, multiple sclerosis, inflammatory bowel disease, rheumatoid arthritis, and psoriasis.[8,14]

   b. **Discuss the sociodemographics of individuals affected by this disease (i.e., age, gender, race, geographic location, other risk factors):**

   Although people of all ages are at risk of developing AA, it typically originates in those aged 25–36. Children may be diagnosed with AA at 5–10 years of age, but such cases are more prevalent with serious forms, such as alopecia universalis.[8] Among diagnosed individuals, almost twice as many women than men have AA, which may be attributed to its autoimmune nature.[16]

The incidence, prevalence, and time since onset of AA are highest in North America and southern Latin America and lowest in North Africa, the Middle East, and South Asia. Additionally, the sociodemographic index has a positive correlation with the number of cases of AA.[16] In the United States, there is a higher risk of AA in African Americans than in whites or Asians.[17]

Many environmental factors affect the development and disease course of AA, including stress, infection, vaccinations, medications, and diet.[8,14] Genetic factors also play a role in the development of AA. According to the National Alopecia Areata Registry, the human leukocyte antigen class II (HLA-D) region on chromosome 6 has the strongest correlation with gene regulation and susceptibility of AA. Though further research is needed to establish the correlation between specific genetic markers and AA, many identical twin, sibling, and familial studies confirm the overall connection between AA and a family history.[8]

8. Discuss the pathogenesis of this disease.

Hair follicles in the anagen (growing) phase are immune privileged, meaning that they are protected from the host immune system, analogous to the anterior chamber of the eyes, the testes, and the uterus while pregnant.[12] In AA, the immune privilege is damaged,[6] which is seen by an increased level of adhesion molecules and major histocompatibility complex (MHC) class I and II,[18] resulting in a surge of lymphocytes entering the hair follicles.[19] These lymphocytes attack anagen hair follicles, abruptly inducing them into the catagen phase.[12,14]

Innate and acquired immunity interact with specific genetic driving factors to drive an interferon-gamma (IFN-γ),[18,19] T-helper 17 (Th17), and B-cell activating factor (BAFF) inflammatory response.[20,21] Cytokines, such as IFN-γ and interleukin (IL)-15, contribute greatly to the inflammation and use secondary messengers, including Janus kinases (JAKs), to further the response.[22] Additionally, the downregulation of regulatory T cells (Tregs) is implicated in AA, as Tregs typically destroy self-reactive T cells by producing natural anti-inflammatory cytokines—transforming growth factor-β (TGF-β) and IL-10.[20] The inflammation not only terminates the growth of the anagen phase but also weakens the hair shaft, resulting in a narrow exclamation point hair.[12] Nail changes, such as nail pitting and longitudinal striations, may also be seen in patients with AA due to the interactions with Th17.[8,23]

9. **What is the clinical presentation of this disease (i.e., grade, stage, sub-types) (Table 10.2)?**

    Classically, AA presents as an acute-onset inflammatory loss of hair in discrete, non-scarring areas on the scalp. Typically, patients report no symptoms, but it is possible to experience itching or tingling prior to the initial loss of hair. In extreme cases, patients can lose all hair on the scalp (alopecia totalis) or body (alopecia universalis).[1] Clinically, when examined with trichoscopy, the affected patches will reveal exclamation point hairs, broken hairs, and yellow dots.[2,12] Also, the patient's nails may present with longitudinal striations, pitting, and ridging.[8,23]

Table 10.2   Types of Alopecia Areata

CLASSIFICATION	CHARACTERISTICS
Alopecia totalis[8]	• Advanced form of AA that results in complete or almost complete loss of scalp hair
Alopecia universalis[8]	• Complete or almost complete hair loss of all bodily surfaces, including eyebrows, eyelashes, chest hair, axillary hair, and pubic hair
Alopecia incognita[8,24]	• Sudden-onset, diffuse, and complete hair loss mainly present in young women • Clinically mimics telogen effluvium
Ophiasis[8]	• Hair loss in the shape of a wave or band-like pattern at the edge of the hairline • Occurs at the perimeter of the temporal and occipital bones
Canities subita[8]	• Abrupt incident of widespread alopecia accompanying graying seemingly "overnight," likely due to the predilection of pigmented hair loss • Also known as Marie Antoinette syndrome

AA: Alopecia areata

10. **Discuss treatment options (Table 10.3).**

    As AA typically recurs, treatment is not considered to be an eternal solution; however, it can stop the advancement of disease and promote hair return.[25] As treatment options are discussed, it is important to treat both psychological and physical aspects of AA patients.[26] There are currently two Food and Drug Administration (FDA)–approved systemic treatments, a few commonly used treatments, and numerous investigational treatments for AA (Table 10.3).[22,27]

    Although the disease course and treatment efficacy of each patient are uncertain, there are influences that negatively impact prognosis, including hairless patches present for over a year, prepubertal loss of hair, positive family history, positive history of atopy, presentation of nail changes, additional autoimmune disorders, and Down's syndrome.[6,18] Additionally, alopecia totalis, alopecia universalis, and ophiasis have a worse prognosis.[18] However, sparse, well-circumscribed patches of AA carry the best prognosis, with approximately half of patients witnessing regrowth in a year.[6]

Table 10.3 Treatment Options for Alopecia Areata

TREATMENT	MECHANISM OF ACTION	NOTES
Baricitinib[22]	A reversible inhibitor of JAK 1 and 2 that disrupts inflammatory cytokine cascades	• Adverse effects: acne, upper respiratory tract infections, urinary tract infections, and increased creatine kinase levels • Taken by mouth • FDA-approved
Ritlecitinib[27]	A JAK 3 and tyrosine kinase inhibitor	• Adverse effects: appendicitis, upper respiratory tract infections, sepsis • Oral administration • FDA-approved
Topical and intralesional corticosteroids[22]	Decreases inflammation	• Adverse effects include cutaneous atrophy • Topical corticosteroids used when patient cannot endure intralesional corticosteroids • Not FDA-approved
Immunotherapy[19,26]	Induces antigenic competition, resulting in allergic contact dermatitis as CD8+ T cells attack the epidermis rather than the hair follicles	• Drugs include dinitrochlorobenzene (DCNB), squaric acid dibutylester (SADBE), and diphenylcyclopropenone (DPCP) • Adverse effects include erythema, pruritus, urticaria, dermatitis, and blistering • Not FDA-approved

AA: alopecia areata; **CD8+:** cluster of differentiation 8; **JAK:** Janus kinase

11. **Other important questions/details:**
    Comorbidities
    AA, while not a deadly condition, may be disfiguring and is associated with substantial emotional and psychological comorbidity; patients with AA often suffer from depression and anxiety disorders.[28] The severe consequence of AA on patients' quality of life and self-esteem can be just as devastating as the hair loss itself.[12]

    AA is associated with increased risk for other autoimmune diseases, particularly systemic lupus erythematosus, type 1 diabetes mellitus, psoriasis, rheumatoid arthritis, thyroid conditions, vitiligo, multiple sclerosis, and inflammatory bowel disease.[8,14] Additionally, AA patients are frequently diagnosed with atopic dermatitis, allergic rhinitis, asthma, vitamin D deficiency, and anemia.[8,29]

References

1. Pinto AC, Andrade TC, Brito FF, Silva GV, Cavalcante ML, Martelli AC. Trichotillomania: A case report with clinical and dermatoscopic differential diagnosis with alopecia areata. *An Bras Dermatol*. 2017;92(1):118–120.
2. Amer M, Helmy A, Amer A. Trichoscopy as a useful method to differentiate tinea capitis from alopecia areata in children at Zagazig University Hospitals. *Int J Dermatol*. 2017;56(1):116–120.

3. Heath CR, Usatine RP. Tinea capitis. *J Fam Pract.* 2022;71(8):370–371. doi:10.12788/jfp.0493

4. Lin Y-T, Li Y-C. The dermoscopic comma zigzag and bar code-like hairs: Markers of fungal infection of the hair follicles. *Dermatologica Sinica*:160–163. doi:10.1016/j.dsi.2013.09.010

5. McElwee KJ, Shapiro JS. Promising therapies for treating and/or preventing androgenic alopecia. *Skin Therapy Lett.* 2012;17(6):1–4.

6. Messenger AG. Alopecia areata: Clinical manifestations and diagnosis. In: Post TW, ed. *UpToDate*. Waltham, MA: UpToDate; 2021. Accessed February 7, 2023. Available from www.uptodate.com/contents/alopecia-areata-clinical-manifestations-and-diagnosis?search=alopecia%20areata&source=search_result&selectedTitle=2~76&usage_type=default&display_rank=2#H17.

7. Kamyab K, Rezvani M, Seirafi H, et al. Distinguishing immunohistochemical features of alopecia areata from androgenic alopecia. *J Cosmet Dermatol.* 2019;18(1):422–426.

8. Pratt CH, King LE, Jr., Messenger AG, Christiano AM, Sundberg JP. Alopecia areata. *Nat Rev Dis Primers.* 2017;3:17011.

9. Heath CR, Usatine RP. Central centrifugal cicatricial alopecia. *J Fam Pract.* 2022;71(3): E13–E14.

10. Mubki T, Rudnicka L, Olszewska M, Shapiro J. Evaluation and diagnosis of the hair loss patient: Part I. History and clinical examination. *J Am Acad Dermatol.* 2014;71(3):415. e1–415.e15.

11. Hughes EC, Saleh D. Telogen effluvium. In: *StatPearls*. Treasure Island, FL: StatPearls Publishing; 2022.

12. Strazzulla LC, Wang EHC, Avila L, et al. Alopecia areata: Disease characteristics, clinical evaluation, and new perspectives on pathogenesis. *J Am Acad Dermatol.* 2018;78(1):1–12.

13. Lima CDS, Lemes LR, Melo DF. Yellow dots in trichoscopy: Relevance, clinical significance and peculiarities. *An Bras Dermatol.* 2017;92(5):724–726.

14. Darwin E, Hirt PA, Fertig R, Doliner B, Delcanto G, Jimenez JJ. Alopecia areata: Review of epidemiology, clinical features, pathogenesis, and new treatment options. *Int J Trichology.* 2018;10(2):51–60.

15. Whiting DA. Histopathologic features of alopecia areata: A new look. *Arch Dermatol.* 2003;139(12):1555–1559.

16. Jang H, Park S, Kim MS, et al. Global, regional and national burden of alopecia areata and its associated diseases, 1990–2019: A systematic analysis of the Global Burden of Disease Study 2019. *Eur J Clin Invest.* 2023;e13958.

17. Lee H, Jung SJ, Patel AB, Thompson JM, Qureshi A, Cho E. Racial characteristics of alopecia areata in the United States. *J Am Acad Dermatol.* 2020;83(4):1064–1070.

18. Sterkens A, Lambert J, Bervoets A. Alopecia areata: A review on diagnosis, immunological etiopathogenesis and treatment options. *Clin Exp Med.* 2021;21(2):215–230.

19. Mahasaksiri T, Kositkuljorn C, Anuntrangsee T, Suchonwanit P. Application of topical immunotherapy in the treatment of alopecia areata: A review and update. *Drug Des Devel Ther.* 2021;15:1285–1298.

20. Elela MA, Gawdat HI, Hegazy RA, et al. B cell activating factor and T-helper 17 cells: Possible synergistic culprits in the pathogenesis of alopecia areata. *Arch Dermatol Res.* 2016;308(2):115–121.

21. Atwa MA, Youssef N, Bayoumy NM. T-helper 17 cytokines (interleukins 17, 21, 22, and 6, and tumor necrosis factor-alpha) in patients with alopecia areata: Association with clinical type and severity. *Int J Dermatol.* 2016;55(6):666–672.

22. King B, Ohyama M, Kwon O, et al. Two phase 3 trials of baricitinib for alopecia areata. *N Engl J Med.* 2022;386(18):1687–1699.

23. Forouzan P, Cohen PR. Systemic lupus erythematosus presenting as alopecia areata. *Cureus.* 2020;12(6):e8724.

24. Molina L, Donati A, Valente NS, Romiti R. Alopecia areata incognita. *Clinics (Sao Paulo)*. 2011;66(3):513–515.

25. Lai VWY, Chen G, Gin D, Sinclair R. Systemic treatments for alopecia areata: A systematic review. *Australas J Dermatol*. 2019;60(1):e1–e13.

26. Messenger AG. Alopecia areata: Management. In: Post TW, ed. *UpToDate*. Waltham, MA: UpToDate; 2022. Accessed February 9, 2023. Available from www.uptodate.com/contents/alopecia-areata-management?search=alopecia%20areat&source=search_result&selectedTitle=1~76&usage_type=default&display_rank=1.

27. Pfizer. LITFULO™ (ritlecitinib) medication page. *Pfizer Medical Information—US*. Accessed November 24, 2023. Available from: www.pfizermedicalinformation.com/litfulo.

28. Shapiro J. Current treatment of alopecia areata. *J Investig Dermatol Symp Proc*. 2013;16(1):S42–S44.

29. Miller R, Conic RZ, Bergfeld W, Mesinkovska NA. Prevalence of comorbid conditions and sun-induced skin cancers in patients with alopecia areata. *J Investig Dermatol Symp Proc*. 2015;17(2):61–62.

11

DIFFUSE, ERYTHEMATOUS PATCHES AND PLAQUES WITH MILD LICHENIFICATION

VARUN K. RANPARIYA AND CRISTIAN C. RIVIS

A 37-year-old white female patient with a history of anxiety and migraines presents to the clinic with a 6-month history of plaques affecting the palmar aspects of both hands (Figure 11.1). The plaques are more significant on her dominant hand. They have ill-defined borders and show erythema, scaling, fissures, crusting, and areas of lichenification. She reports stinging, burning, and itching. The patient states she has tried using moisturizers and hydrocortisone cream, but they only provide temporary relief. She denies any allergies or previous history of skin conditions. She reports she works as a chef.

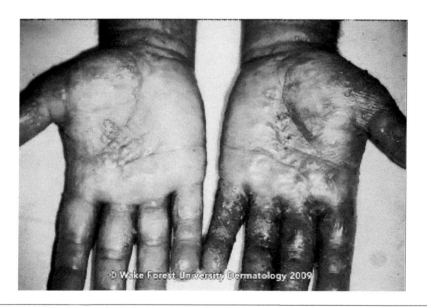

Figure 11.1 Patient presentation.

1. **How would you describe the lesion?**
   The lesion is present on the palmar aspect of both hands, but more significant on her right hand. It is characterized as diffuse and poorly defined, erythematous

DOI: 10.1201/9781003437987-11

patches and plaques with areas of lichenification. There are areas of hyperkeratosis with fissures as well as scaling and crusting.

2. What are the differential diagnoses (Table 11.1)?

Table 11.1 Differential Diagnoses for Diffuse, Erythematous Patches and Plaques with Mild Lichenification

DIAGNOSIS	COMMENTS
Palmoplantar psoriasis	Palmoplantar psoriasis frequently presents with lesions at distant sites such as the elbows and knees. In addition, nail psoriasis is commonly present. The lack of these concomitant signs makes this diagnosis less likely.[1]
Dyshidrotic eczema (hand eczema)	Dyshidrotic eczema can be differentiated from other conditions causing erythematous patches by the presence of vesicles and bullae on palms and soles. These lesions usually involve the palms and the lateral and medial aspects of the fingers.[2]
Atopic dermatitis	In adults, atopic dermatitis typically presents as thickened plaques with lichenification and scale with pruritus. Lesions are usually at flexural folds, eyelids, forehead, cheeks, and perioral region. Atopic dermatitis primarily appears on the volar wrists and dorsum of the hands. The disease has a chronic course with temporary remission in the summer. Most patients will have a personal or family history of atopy that supports a diagnosis of atopic dermatitis.[3]
Allergic contact dermatitis (ACD)	ACD often presents as a well-demarcated, pruritic, eczematous eruption. It can be acute or chronic. The chronic form typically presents with lichenification or scaly plaques. However, since the offending allergen could be a shampoo or lotion, which contacts the whole body, patchy or diffuse lesion distributions can be seen. Given the similar clinical presentation of ICD and ACD, especially the chronic forms, patch testing is often used to make a diagnosis of ACD.[2]
Irritant contact dermatitis (ICD)	The clinical presentation of ICD is multifaceted, shaped by the specific irritants, host characteristics, duration of exposure, and environmental conditions. ICD is an umbrella diagnosis encompassing diverse subtypes, each characterized by certain offending agents, patterns of exposure, and clinical manifestations. The general mechanisms of injury involve irritants damaging cell membranes, altering epidermal keratins, and exerting direct cytotoxic effects. ICD reactions are non-immune-mediated, a feature distinguishing them from ACD. Acute exposure typically results in erythema, burning sensations, scaling, pruritus, vesiculation, and epidermal erosions, while chronic exposures may lead to hyperkeratosis, lichenification, and fissuring of affected areas. In the absence of a clear exposure history, ICD can be a diagnosis of exclusion given its myriad presentations. While not definitive or exclusive, ICD tends to present more frequently with burning, and ACD more frequently with pruritus. Patch testing is often performed to rule out ACD.[2]

3. What is the most likely diagnosis?

The most likely diagnosis for this patient is chronic irritant contact dermatitis (ICD).

4. What is the next best step?

The initial clinical workup should include a thorough skin examination and history. Exploring the patient's daily activities, workplace environment, hand washing habits, and accidental exposures can help identify a causative irritant. However, the irritant, as well as the concentration and duration of exposure, are often unknown. Therefore, ICD is a diagnosis of exclusion.[2] Patch testing and histological examination may be useful in making a diagnosis.

5. **What are the most appropriate diagnostic modalities (i.e., labs, biopsies, scrapings, histological findings)?**

   Patch testing is the most commonly used diagnostic modality for ICD. In the case of a localized dermatitis, it will be difficult to differentiate between a diagnosis of ICD and allergic contact dermatitis (ACD). There is a high degree of similarity between ICD and ACD in regard to clinical appearance, histopathology, and immunohistology. Therefore, in order to exclude ACD, a patch test must be performed.[2]

   Patch testing is a diagnostic tool that tests a variety of allergens by inducing a delayed-type hypersensitivity reaction in pre-sensitized individuals. It is the gold standard for diagnosing ACD. Patch testing is indicated when a contact dermatitis is suspected. This includes acute or chronic dermatitis that may manifest with erythema, edema, weeping, crusting, scaling, hyperkeratosis, and lichenification. Other indications include chronic dermatitis that is not improving with treatment or previously well-controlled dermatitis that is worsening. While there are thousands of potential allergens, the ones chosen tend to be based on history and examination. The American Contact Dermatitis Society and the European Contact Dermatitis Society have both created a baseline or standard series of allergens to optimize patch testing results. These panels are dynamic—they are continuously evaluated and can be modified. If the patient's history suggests exposure to certain allergens, they should also be added to the testing panel.

   Patch testing is usually performed in a general clinic setting and requires three office visits. Testing is typically done on the upper back, as it provides enough surface area for application. If the back is not suitable or additional space is required, the upper arms and thighs may be used. It is recommended to avoid patch testing during acute flare of dermatitis, as it can result in false-positive reactions. The first visit, or day 0, is to place the patch test. On day 2 (48 hours), allergens should be removed, and a preliminary patch test read is taken 15 minutes after removal. A final reading is taken on day 3 (72 hours) or day 4 (96 hours); this final reading time frame varies among different testing centers. Patch test reading is based on morphology that places reactions into three categories: questionable reactions, irritant reactions, and clear positive reactions. The most common irritant reaction features include pustular, purpuric, glazed, or scorched epidermal changes. Clear positive reactions are graded based on the presence of erythema, induration, papules, and vesicles. The most challenging part of patch testing is the process of interpreting the results. Although a patient may test positive, this does not necessarily result in a diagnosis of ACD. The patient's clinical manifestation and history must be examined to establish the relevance of a positive patch test reaction. If the allergen that tested positive can be identified in the patient's history or environment, probable relevance can be assigned. True relevance is established if clinical outcomes correlate with adequate allergen avoidance.[4]

6. **What would you expect to find in the histopathologic analysis?**

   Although not performed often, a skin biopsy may be helpful when the differential is broader than just dermatitis.[5] It can be used to differentiate ICD from psoriasis, tinea, cutaneous T-cell lymphoma, or other types of inflammatory dermatoses.

   Based on the stage and severity of the ICD, the histologic features will be different. The diversity in the histologic features of ICD can be attributed to different ways different chemicals interact with the skin. Mild spongiosis, intraepidermal vesicle or bullae, and necrosis of keratinocytes are characteristic of acute ICD.[6] Chronic ICD is characterized by hyperkeratosis, parakeratosis, acanthosis, spongiosis, and exocytosis.[7]

7. **Discuss the epidemiology of this disease**.

   a. **Discuss the incidence and prevalence:**

   ICD is the most common form of contact dermatitis and represents between 70% and 80% of all occupational skin disorders. According to a survey by the National Institutes of Occupational Safety and Health in 2010, the overall prevalence of dermatitis was 10.2%. The survey utilized a sample cohort of 27,157 individuals to represent the U.S. adult population. The incidence of occupational contact dermatitis has a range of 50–70 cases/100,000 workers per year.[2]

   b. **Discuss the sociodemographics of individuals affected by this disease (i.e., age, gender, race, geographic location, other risk factors):**

   Many different sociodemographic characteristics can predispose an individual to develop ICD. Age, sex, site of exposure, and pre-existing skin diseases are important predisposing characteristics. Regarding age, infants and the elderly are at an increased risk of being affected by ICD due to their less effective epidermal barrier. Furthermore, ICD is likely to manifest with more severe symptoms in those patients. Women are also more often affected than men. ICD is more likely to develop on body parts that are more often exposed to irritants. Therefore, hand involvement is seen in about 80% of patients. Prior history of skin diseases is a significant risk factor for occupational dermatitis—13.5 times greater risk in those with atopic dermatitis. "Wet work" occupations, such as food handlers, health care workers, cleaners, housekeepers and mechanical industry workers, tend to have excessive exposure to water, soaps, and detergents. These are common causes of ICD, and therefore individuals with these occupations are at an increased risk of developing it.[2]

8. **Discuss the pathogenesis of this disease.**

The pathogenesis of ICD is not completely understood. However, it is thought that multiple mechanisms may be involved depending on the irritant. These mechanisms include disruption of the epidermal barrier, damage of keratinocyte cell membranes, cytotoxic effects on keratinocytes, cytokine release from keratinocytes, and activation of innate immunity. Furthermore, the mechanisms responsible for acute and chronic ICD are different. Direct cytotoxic damage to keratinocytes is seen in acute reactions. Chronic reactions occur due to slower damage to cell membranes, which occurs due to repeated exposures to solvents and surfactants that remove surface lipids and water-retaining substances.[2]

The initiating event of acute ICD is thought to be disruption of the epidermal barrier or the stratum corneum. Once an irritant penetrates the barrier, mild damage or stress to keratinocytes results. This in turn releases mediators of inflammation with resultant T-cell activation. These mediators include cytokines such as interleukin (IL)-1α, IL-1-β, IL-6, and tumor necrosis factor-α (TNF-α). TNF-α and IL-1α are the primary mediators and are responsible for inducing the production of other cytokines, chemokines, and adhesion molecules. A predominant feature of ICD is the expression of intercellular adhesion molecule-1 (ICAM-1). This molecule is upregulated by TNF-α, IL-6, and IL-1-β.[2]

In most cases of ICD, the lesions will resolve despite continued exposure due to a process known as the "hardening phenomenon." Although the exact mechanism is unknown, there are a few theories to explain the phenomenon. This includes irritant-induced changes in skin morphology and barrier function that may make it more difficult for the irritant to penetrate. In addition, changes in skin permeability and vascular reactivity may allow for faster removal of irritants.[8]

If ICD cannot be resolved, chronic ICD will develop. As a result of damage to the stratum corneum lipids, there is loss of cohesion or corneocytes, desquamation, and an increase in transepidermal water loss (TEWL). The increase in TEWL triggers restoration of the cutaneous barrier via the promotion of lipid synthesis, keratinocyte proliferation, and transient hyperkeratosis. In the setting of damage with a solvent, this restorative mechanism is disrupted. There is blockage of water evaporation, which halts lipid synthesis and barrier recovery. Chronic exposure results in increased epidermal turnover, manifesting as a chronic ICD.[2]

9. **What is the clinical presentation of this disease (i.e., grade, stage, subtypes)?**

Multiple variants of ICD have been described (Table 11.2); however, the most common forms encountered are acute and chronic ICD.

Table 11.2 Clinical Variations of ICD[2]

TYPE OF ICD	DESCRIPTION
Acute ICD	Due to an acute exposure to potent irritants and is usually accidental. Presents within minutes to hours after exposure. Lesions have sharply demarcated borders and include erythema, edema, bullae, and possibly necrosis. Patients may feel burning, stinging, and soreness. Healing begins soon after removal of irritant.
Acute delayed ICD	Delayed inflammatory response seen in certain irritants (e.g., anthralin, benzalkonium chloride, and ethylene oxide). Inflammation is not seen until 8–24 hours or more after exposure. Patients usually experience burning as well as sensitivity to touch and water.
Irritant reaction ICD	Characterized by scaling, redness, vesicles, pustules, and erosions. The lesion often begins under occlusive jewelry (e.g., rings) and then spreads. Seen in individuals frequently exposed to wet chemical environments. May result in chronic ICD is exposure is prolonged.
Cumulative ICD	Also known as chronic ICD. Lesions are less sharply demarcated and usually involve lichenification and hyperkeratosis. Xerosis, erythema, and vesicles may also be present. Pruritus and pain are symptoms of cumulative ICD.
Asteatotic dermatitis	Also known as asteatotic eczema, it is characterized by dry skin with ichthyosiform scale and patches of superficially cracked skin with intense pruritus. It is primarily seen during the dry winter months and in elderly individuals who frequently bathe without remoisturizing.
Traumatic ICD	Characterized by eczematous lesions with persistent redness, infiltration, scale, and fissures at the affected site. It most commonly presents on the hands. Traumatic ICD may develop after trauma such as lacerations, burns, or even acute ICD.
Pustular and acneiform ICD	Acne-like lesions that result from exposure to irritants such as metals, croton oil, tars, greases, and metal working fluids. Pustules that develop are transient and "sterile."
Non-erythematous ICD	Subclinical form of ICD, in which changes to the stratum corneum function may be apparent, but without a clinical correlate.
Subjective or sensory ICD	Symptoms of stinging or burning in the absence of visible signs of irritation. This form of ICD can be caused by exposure to propylene glycol, hydroxy acids, benzoic acid, and ethanol as well as topical medications such as lactic acid, azelaic acid, benzoyl peroxide, mequinol, and tretinoin.
Airborne ICD	Usually develops in irritant-exposed parts of the face and periorbital regions. There is usually involvement of the upper eyelids, philtrum, and submental regions. Exposure to floating dusts, fibers, and volatile solvents and sprays can cause airborne ICD.
Frictional ICD	Results from repeated low-grade frictional trauma. It presents with hyperkeratosis, acanthosis, and lichenification.

ICD: Irritant contact dermatitis

10. Discuss treatment options.

The primary treatment is avoiding the causative irritants. Irritants should be identified, and efforts should be made to substitute or reduce exposure to them. Preventative measures that can be taken in the workplace include using protective creams (for intact skin), mild cleaning agents (to remove irritants), and emollients or moisturizers (to enhance barrier function).[2]

Treating skin inflammation and restoring epidermal barrier function involve a combination therapy of topical corticosteroids and emollients/moisturizers. Although often used in clinical practice, treating ICD with topical corticosteroids has been controversial. Conflicting results have been provided from experimental studies. The primary factor driving topical corticosteroid use in ICD is their anti-inflammatory properties. Given the lack of proven benefit, the adverse effects of using topical corticosteroids should be weighed against the potential benefits on a case-by-case basis. Choosing the appropriate topical corticosteroid is dependent on the location and severity of the ICD.[2]

Additional first-line therapies include emollients and barrier creams. Several studies have shown lipid-rich moisturizers are effective in reducing erythema, scaling, and TEWL in experimentally induced skin irritation. Therefore, in addition to being used as a preventative measure, they are also beneficial in treating ICD. When present on the skin, they can decrease irritation and improve skin barrier function. Emollients and moisturizers should be applied liberally multiple times a day.[9]

Additional therapeutic modalities may be useful in stubborn cases. For those with chronic dermatitis that does not respond to any other forms of therapy, narrowband ultraviolet B or photochemical therapy irradiation may be considered. Adjunctive use of systemic retinoids (e.g., acitretin and alitretinoin) or systemic immunomodulators (e.g., methotrexate and cyclosporine) should be considered in those with a combination of dermatitis and psoriasis or hyperkeratotic palmoplantar dermatitis stemming from frictional or chronic ICD.[2]

11. **Other important questions/details:**
    What is the prognosis?
    As mentioned before, ICD resolves via "hardening" in many individuals. However, the timing of this phenomenon varies from person to person. For some, the ICD will progress to a chronic phrase. Those with a poorer prognosis have been associated with a history of atopy, female gender, and the presence of ACD. Early diagnosis, treatment, and patient education can potentially improve prognosis.[2]

References

1. Miceli A, Schmieder GJ. *Palmoplantar Psoriasis*. Treasure Island, FL: StatPearls Publishing; 2019.
2. Bolognia J, Schaffer JV, Cerroni L. *Dermatology*. 4th ed. Elsevier; 2017.
3. Pugliarello S, Cozzi A, Gisondi P, Girolomoni G. Phenotypes of atopic dermatitis. *JDDG: Journal der Deutschen Dermatologischen Gesellschaft*. 2011;9(1):12–20.
4. Uyesugi BA, Sheehan MP. Patch testing pearls. *Clin Rev Allergy Immunol*. 2019;56(1): 110–118.
5. Frings VG, Boer-Auer A, Breuer K. Histomorphology and immunophenotype of eczematous skin lesions revisited-skin biopsies are not reliable in differentiating allergic contact dermatitis, irritant contact dermatitis, and atopic dermatitis. *Am J Dermatopathol*. 2018;40(1):7–16.

6. Willis CM, Stephens CJ, Wilkinson JD. Epidermal damage induced by irritants in man: A light and electron microscopic study. *J Invest Dermatol.* 1989;93(5):695–699.
7. Willis CM. Histopathology of irritant contact dermatitis. In: *Irritant Dermatitis.* Berlin, Heidelberg: Springer; 2006.
8. Watkins SA, Maibach HI. The hardening phenomenon in irritant contact dermatitis: An interpretative update. *Contact Dermatitis.* 2009;60(3):123–130.
9. Lebwohl M, Heymann WR, Berth-Jones J, Coulson I, eds., *Treatment of Skin Disease: Comprehensive Therapeutic Strategies.* 5th ed. Elsevier; 2018.

12
ITCHY, RED SPOTS ON TORSO AND ARMS

VERONICA EMMERICH AND SOFIA PEDROZA

A 34-year-old female with a history of endometriosis and acute simple cystitis presents to the clinic for evaluation of a new rash on her trunk and arms (Figure 12.1). The patient first noticed the rash 2 days ago, and she reports that the rash appeared on her chest before spreading to her arms. Otherwise, she feels well. She is currently taking a 7-day course of cefpodoxime. The rash is red, raised, and mildly pruritic. She took diphenhydramine last night to relieve the itch but has not tried any other treatments. The patient works as a preschool teacher.

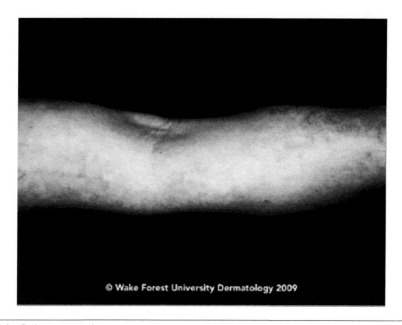

© Wake Forest University Dermatology 2009

Figure 12.1 Patient presentation.

1. **How would you describe the lesion?**
   The lesions are diffuse, bright red macules and papules 1–5 mm in diameter symmetrically distributed across the patient's torso and arms. There are large areas of confluence across the chest and abdomen.

DOI: 10.1201/9781003437987-12

2. What are the differential diagnoses (Table 12.2)?

Table 12.1   Differential Diagnoses for Itchy, Red Spots on Torso and Arms

DIAGNOSIS	COMMENTS
Viral exanthem	Viral exanthems are generalized eruptions caused by a vascular response to viral infection. Although viral exanthems are not specific to any virus, they are most associated with rubeola (measles), rubella (German measles), herpesvirus type 6 (roseola), and parvovirus B19. While viral exanthems do occur in adults, they are more common among children and are typically preceded by constitutional symptoms such as fever.[1] Some viral exanthems exhibit characteristic features: • In rubeola and rubella, the rash typically starts on the head before proceeding inferiorly. In rubeola, the rash tends to coalesce on the face and trunk but remains discrete elsewhere.[1] • The rash of HHV-6 (roseola) occurs primarily in children under the age of 2 and is preceded by a high-grade fever.[2] • Parvovirus B19 causes a "slapped cheek" rash (erythema infectiosum) followed by reticulated erythema on the trunk and extremities.[1]
Exanthematous drug eruption	Exanthematous drug eruptions, also known as morbilliform or maculopapular drug eruptions, are the most common drug-induced skin eruptions. They present with symmetrically distributed, pruritic, red-to-pink macules or papules that may coalesce, forming plaques. Most exanthematous drug eruptions evolve rapidly after initial exposure to the offending agent, reaching maximal severity approximately 2 days into the course of the drug. This time course may vary from several hours to several days depending on whether it is a first-time exposure to the offending agent or a repeated exposure.[2]
Toxic erythema	Toxic erythemas are typically due to bacterial infection, especially group A streptococci and *Staphylococcus aureus*. Scarlet fever, SSSS, and TSS are toxic erythemas caused by a cutaneous response to toxins elaborated by these two bacteria. These rashes are characterized by fever and a sandpaper-like rash that is accentuated in flexural folds, often followed by desquamation. Patients will have a history of a sore throat (scarlet fever), local infection (SSSS), tampon use (TSS), or recent surgery (TSS).[1]
DRESS syndrome	DRESS syndrome is a severe drug reaction characterized by a cutaneous eruption with multiorgan involvement.[3] This reaction typically occurs 2–8 weeks following exposure to the inciting agent and commonly includes fever, lymphadenopathy, hematologic abnormalities (eosinophilia, abnormal erythrocyte morphology), and abnormal liver function tests.[3,4] DRESS syndrome is historically associated with phenytoin and has a 10% mortality rate, which is often due to renal or hepatic involvement.[3]
Syphilis	The rash of secondary syphilis commonly presents as scaling papules and plaques, and the patient may recall a primary chancre. A generalized eruption with palmar and plantar involvement is suggestive of syphilis. Systemic symptoms such as fever and myalgia are usually present.[1]

DRESS: Drug reaction with eosinophilia and systemic symptoms; **HHV-6:** human herpesvirus type 6; **SSSS:** staphylococcal scalded skin syndrome; **TSS:** toxic shock syndrome.

3. What is the most likely diagnosis?

The most likely diagnosis in this patient is an exanthematous drug eruption.

4. What is the next best step?

The next best step in management of these multiple lesions suspicious for a drug eruption is to elucidate a detailed history from the patient to establish a timeline between initiation of a drug and the onset of the eruption.

Reviewing medical records may also be helpful. Once the offending agent is identified, it should be discontinued. In patients who are hospitalized or taking multiple drugs, it may be difficult to identify the causative agent, in which case the number of drugs being administered should be minimized. Beta-lactam antibiotics, sulfonamides, antiepileptics, and non-corticosteroid anti-inflammatory drugs are frequently implicated.[1]

After discontinuing the drug, therapy is symptomatic. Antihistamines may be prescribed to treat pruritus, and moisturizing lotions may be helpful if desquamation is present. Severe pruritus may warrant a short course of systemic corticosteroids.[1]

5. **What are the most appropriate diagnostic modalities (i.e., labs, biopsies, scrapings, histological findings)?**
   Exanthematous drug eruption is a clinical diagnosis that relies on knowing the time between the initiation of the drug and the onset of the eruption. No laboratory tests will confirm the diagnosis, and a biopsy is not recommended.

6. **What would you expect to find in the histopathologic analysis?**
   Histopathologic analysis of an exanthematous drug eruption will reveal a superficial, perivascular, mononuclear infiltrate, typically composed of CD3+ T cells, neutrophils, and eosinophils. CD4+ T cells predominate in the perivascular dermis, but CD4+ and CD8+ T cells are equally distributed at the dermo-epidermal junction.[5] The epidermis will appear normal.[1] However, these findings are not specific.[6]

7. **Discuss the epidemiology of this disease**.
   a. **Discuss the incidence and prevalence:**
      There are limited data on cutaneous drug reactions outside of the hospital setting; in hospitalized patients, cutaneous reactions occur in up to 8% of patients. Most of these reactions are exanthematous, or morbilliform, eruptions.[6] Exanthematous drug eruptions make up approximately 95% of cutaneous drug eruptions, making this condition the most common of cutaneous drug reactions.[7]

   b. **Discuss the sociodemographics of individuals affected by this disease (i.e., age, gender, race, geographic location, other risk factors):**
      Cutaneous drug reactions may occur in any individual taking any drug. However, females, immunosuppressed patients, patients with dermatomyositis, and carriers of certain human leukocyte antigen (HLA) alleles are at increased risk for exanthematous eruptions. Individuals with human immunodeficiency virus (HIV), for example, are at 10- to 50-fold increased risk for a drug reaction to sulfamethoxazole.[6]

8. **Discuss the pathogenesis of this disease**.
   Many cutaneous drug reactions, including exanthematous drug eruptions, are due to a delayed (type IV) hypersensitivity reaction.[2] Antigen-presenting cells present either the drug or its metabolite to naïve T cells; these T cells then

proliferate and infiltrate the skin, where they produce cytokines and chemo-kines that mediate an inflammatory response. The severity and type of reaction depend on which subset of T cells is predominantly activated.[5]

In exanthematous drug eruptions, cytotoxic CD4+ T cells are dominant and act as effector cells. They migrate to tissues, where they induce apoptosis of keratinocytes via a perforin/granzyme, granulysin, and Fas/FasL-dependent manner.[8] Keratinocytes, which express major histocompatibility class (MHC) II, present the drug or its metabolite and thus are targeted for destruction.[9] Additionally, CD4+ T cells secrete type 1 and type 2 cytokines; in particular, the release of interleukin (IL)-5 contributes to eosinophilia, a common characteristic in drug allergy.[8] The inflammation leads to vasodilation and increased vascular permeability, which result in the blanchable macules and papules characteristic of an exanthematous drug eruption.

9. **What is the clinical presentation of this disease (i.e., grade, stage, subtypes)?**

Exanthematous drug eruption, also known as maculopapular exanthema and morbilliform drug-induced exanthem, involves a maculopapular rash. The first signs of an incoming maculopapular exanthem may be detected as erythema a few hours after initial exposure to the offending agent. The characteristic condition presents approximately 7–10 days into the duration of exposure as erythematous macules and infiltrated papules from 1 to 5 mm in diameter, often accompanied by pruritus and a low-grade fever. These macules and papules may spread across the proximal extremities, trunk, and/or face, typically bilaterally and symmetrically. Exanthems may vary in appearance depending on severity of reaction. Strong reactions may lead to confluent macules and/or papules resulting in erythroderma and plaques. Significant desquamation will occur as the eruption progresses and clears. The condition will typically resolve within 7–14 days after cessation of offending agent exposure.[10,11] Upon re-exposure to the same agent, recurrence of these symptoms may occur sooner, ranging from 6 hours to 7 days.[11]

Differentiating between drug-induced exanthems and viral exanthems based on clinical presentation can be challenging. Exanthematous drug eruptions and viral exanthems produce similar maculopapular rashes accompanied by overlapping symptoms such as fever, pharyngitis, and malaise. The location of spread may appear similarly in both conditions, although viral exanthems may spread predominantly across the face and neck. Additionally, some infections with these accompanying symptoms may be treated with drugs that cause drug-induced exanthems. The resolution of the eruption upon discontinuation of a drug and the reprovocation of the eruption upon readministration of it remain the most definitive indications that the eruption is drug-induced.[2,12] Recent research suggests potential hematological and histological differences between the two types of exanthems that may be useful in confirmation of diagnoses.[12] In this case, the rapid onset of the patient's rash following the use of a cephalosporin makes drug eruption a more likely diagnosis than viral exanthem.

10. **Discuss treatment options**.

Determine the probable causative agent and cease use, then monitor for resolution. Oral antihistamines and corticosteroids may be used to reduce severe symptoms. For example, diphenhydramine, a sedating antihistamine, may be used to decrease severe pruritus associated with the rashes. The desquamation seen in the resolution of the lesions can also cause pruritus that may be relieved using topical corticosteroids such as hydrocortisone and non-sensitizing emollients such as petroleum jelly. Potent topical glucocorticoids also reduce pruritus and the appearance of severe rashes.[13]

11. **Other important questions/details:**

Other types of drug eruptions include acute generalized exanthematous pustulosis (AGEP), lichenoid reaction (LR), erythroderma, and vasculitis (Table 12.2).

Table 12.2 Differential Diagnoses for Non-exanthematous (Morbilliform) Drug Eruption

DIAGNOSIS	COMMENTS
Acute generalized exanthematous pustulosis (AGEP)	AGEP presents as small, sterile pustules distributed across a confluent exanthem or edematous erythema. These pustules may proliferate and merge, becoming large, confluent areas. This frequently appears on areas of the body where skin folds touch, rub, and result in occlusion, such as axillae. Some systemic effects such as fever, leukocytosis with neutrophilia, and eosinophilia may be involved. AGEP typically presents after 1–2 days of antibiotic intake, such as aminopenicillin intake, or up to 11 days for other drugs such as terbinafine.[14]
Erythroderma	Acute erythroderma or exfoliative dermatitis can be caused by infections and drug reactions. It presents as either a morbilliform rash, urticaria, or pustules followed by erythroderma and exfoliative scaling up to 6 days after onset. These symptoms may differ depending on underlying malignancies such as Stevens-Johnson syndrome, causing blisters and/or mucocutaneous lesions.[15]
Lichenoid reaction (LR)	LR presents as small, shiny, raised papules that are a reddish-purple color, localizing especially on the anterior arms, hands, and back. LR can be triggered by medications such as antihistamines and corticosteroids but is still considered a rare condition in response to medications.[16]
Vasculitis	Vasculitis is a less common culprit for drug-associated reactions; however, leukocytoclastic vasculitis is the most commonly seen vasculitis drug eruption. It presents similarly to other types of vasculitis, with petechiae, palpable purpuric eruptions, and/or bullae.[14]

References

1. Marks J, Miller J. *Lookingbill and Marks' Principles of Dermatology*. 6th ed. Elsevier; 2019.
2. Stern RS. Clinical practice: Exanthematous drug eruptions. *N Engl J Med*. 2012;366(26): 2492–2501.
3. Choudhary S, McLeod M, Torchia D, Romanelli P. Drug Reaction with Eosinophilia and Systemic Symptoms (DRESS) syndrome. *J Clin Aesthet Dermatol*. 2013;6(6):31–37.

4. Dorrell DN, Whitaker LF, Anderson KL, Strowd LC. Abnormal erythrocyte morphology in drug reaction with eosinophilia and systemic symptoms. *J Am Acad Dermatol.* 2019;80(4):1159–1160.

5. Rozieres A, Vocanson M, Said BB, Nosbaum A, Nicolas JF. Role of T cells in nonimmediate allergic drug reactions. *Curr Opin Allergy Clin Immunol.* 2009;9(4):305–310.

6. Bolognia J, Schaffer J, Cerroni L. *Dermatology.* 4th ed. Philadelphia: Elsevier; 2018.

7. Washington NR, Petersen K, Petersen M. The clindamycin catastrophe: A case of antibiotic-induced skin eruption. *Clin Pediatr (Phila).* January, 2019;58(1):120–122.

8. Pichler WJ, Adam J, Daubner B, Gentinetta T, Keller M, Yerly D. Drug hypersensitivity reactions: Pathomechanism and clinical symptoms. *Med Clin North Am.* 2010;94(4): 645–664, xv.

9. Pichler WJ, Yawalkar N. Allergic reactions to drugs: involvement of T cells. *Thorax.* 2000;55(Suppl 2):S61–S65.

10. Bircher AJ, Scherer K. Delayed cutaneous manifestations of drug hypersensitivity. *Med Clin North Am.* July, 2010;94(4):711–725, x.

11. Crisafulli G, Franceschini F, Caimmi S, Bottau P, Liotti L, Saretta F, Bernardini R, Cardinale F, Mori F, Caffarelli C. Mild cutaneous reactions to drugs. *Acta Biomed.* January 28, 2019;90(3-S):36–43.

12. Khandpur S, Ahuja R. Drug-induced vs. Viral maculopapular exanthem-resolving the dilemma. *Dermatopathology (Basel).* May 7, 2022;9(2):164–171.

13. Segal AR, Doherty KM, Leggott J, Zlotoff B. Cutaneous reactions to drugs in children. *Pediatrics.* October, 2007;120(4):e1082–e1096.

14. Brockow, K, Ardern-Jones, MR, Mockenhaupt, M, et al. EAACI position paper on how to classify cutaneous manifestations of drug hypersensitivity. *Allergy.* 2019;74:14–27.

15. Tso S, Satchwell F, Moiz H, Hari T, Dhariwal S, Barlow R, Forbat E, Randeva H, Tan YT, Ilchyshyn A, Kwok MM, Barber TM, Thind C, Tso ACY. Erythroderma (exfoliative dermatitis). Part 1: Underlying causes, clinical presentation and pathogenesis. *Clin Exp Dermatol.* August, 2021;46(6):1001–1010.

16. Suryana K. Lichenoid eeaction caused by antihistamines and corticosteroids. *J Asthma Allergy.* June 30, 2020;13:205–211.

13

WELL-DEFINED, CHALKY WHITE MACULES AND PATCHES

ROKSANA HESARI AND CRISTIAN C. RIVIS

A 51-year-old Caucasian female with a past medical history of well-controlled Hashimoto's thyroiditis presents to the clinic reporting the presence of "white spots" on her face, abdomen, and extremities (Figure 13.1). The patient reports that she has had these spots for several years and they do not cause any symptoms. Initially, the spots were small and limited to her face, but over time they have gradually spread across her body and increased in both size and number. She denies any recent trauma

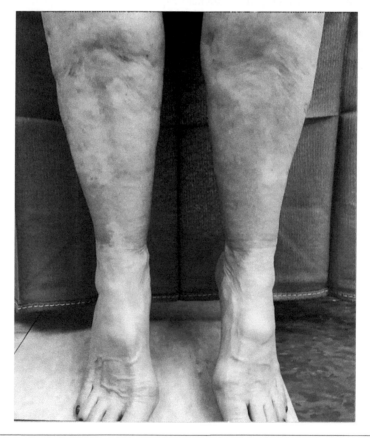

Figure 13.1   Patient presentation

DOI: 10.1201/9781003437987-13

or infection of the affected areas but mentions that her aunt also has similar skin lesions. The patient notes that the spots are more noticeable during summer months after spending time at the beach, especially on days when she forgets to reapply sunscreen. She has attempted to conceal the spots with makeup, as she dislikes their appearance and wishes to know if they can be eliminated entirely.

1. **How would you describe the lesion?**

   The lesions are symmetric, chalky white macules and patches that have well-defined borders with no accompanying erythema or overlying scale.

2. **What are the differential diagnoses (Table 13.1)?**

Table 13.1   Differential Diagnoses for Depigmented Macules and Patches

DIAGNOSIS	COMMENTS
Vitiligo	Vitiligo is a complex acquired skin condition with a multifactorial etiology involving genetic, autoimmune, and environmental factors.[1] Typically patients have one or more symmetrical patches that lack pigmentation bordered by normal skin.[2] These areas of depigmentation frequently grow in size and quantity over time. Family history of similar lesions is common.
Pityriasis alba	Pityriasis alba is a self-limiting condition that usually affects children and adolescents. It is characterized by poorly defined, hypopigmented, dry, scaly macules on the face that may be pruritic.[3] This condition generally resolves on its own within a few months.
Tinea versicolor	Tinea versicolor is a fungal infection (*Malassezia*) that can cause multiple hypopigmented or hyperpigmented macules with a fine scale on the skin. The scale is more apparent upon scratching or stretching the skin.[3] The lesions are typically present on the upper trunk or chest. On Wood's lamp examination, these lesions reveal a golden to yellow-green fluorescent color.[3,4] Lesions suspicious for tinea versicolor can be tested with potassium hydroxide (KOH) preparation, as they will reveal a characteristic spaghetti and meatball appearance of the fungal hyphae and spores.[2] Even after proper treatment, hypopigmentation can persist for months.[3]
Piebaldism	Piebaldism is a rare congenital disorder that presents at birth with depigmented areas on the skin. It is inherited in an autosomal dominant manner and is characterized by an absence of melanocytes in the impacted regions of skin.[5] These patients present with a white forelock and a triangular, amelanotic patch on their forehead.[3]
Tuberculoid leprosy	Tuberculoid leprosy, otherwise known as Hansen's disease, is an acquired chronic granulomatous condition found in endemic areas. The causative agent is *Mycobacterium leprae*, a bacterium that infects the skin and cutaneous nerves in cool areas of the body.[6] In this particular form of leprosy, there are few organisms present in the skin. The lesions are few in number and are described as thin, well-defined, hypopigmented macules and plaques with raised edges. These lesions lack sensation secondary to infection of the peripheral nerves supplying the region.[3,6] Diagnosis can be made with slit skin smears with Ziehl-Neelsen staining and polymerase chain reaction (PCR).[6]
Post-inflammatory hypopigmentation	Post-inflammatory hypopigmentation is the result of an injury or inflammatory skin condition that, once healed, results in the loss of pigmentation to the affected area. Unlike this case, the hypopigmentation seen in this condition is often poorly demarcated and localized.[3,6] Patients will report a history of preceding trauma or inflammation to the affected area.

(Continued)

Table 13.1 (*Continued*)   Differential Diagnoses for Depigmented Macules and Patches

DIAGNOSIS	COMMENTS
Tuberous sclerosis	Tuberous sclerosis is a disease that presents in infancy and is inherited in an autosomal dominant manner. The mutated gene normally codes for a tumor suppressor involved in regulating the growth of cells derived from the ectoderm and mesoderm. The primary clinical manifestations of tuberous sclerosis include the triad of congenital hypomelanotic macules, seizures, and mental retardation.[3,6] The shapes of the white macules are classically described as being polygonal/thumbprint, lance ovate/ash-leaf, or confetti spots. Other skin manifestations in those affected include facial angiofibromas, shagreen patch, and periungual papules/nodules.[6]
Idiopathic guttate hypomelanosis	Idiopathic guttate hypomelanosis is an acquired skin condition that commonly affects elderly individuals with a history of long-term sun exposure.[3] It is characterized by numerous small, hypomelanotic macules measuring between 1 and 5 mm on sun-exposed areas of the body.[2,5] These lesions are asymptomatic and have a smooth surface.[3]
Lichen sclerosus	Lichen sclerosus is an acquired disorder most commonly affecting the anogenital skin of postmenopausal women, although children and males can rarely be affected too. The lesions are sharply defined, hypopigmented papules that coalesce into plaques. Purpura is generally also present, and atrophy occurs. At times, the labia minora and majora fuse. Patients often complain of pain and pruritus of the genitalia; however, in rare cases where extragenital skin is involved, those lesions tend to be asymptomatic. In patients where lichen sclerosus is suspected, biopsy can be diagnostic.[6]

3. **What is the most likely diagnosis?**

Based on the patient's medical history of autoimmune thyroid disease, family history of a similar condition, distinctive cutaneous lesions, and lack of associated symptoms, the most likely diagnosis is vitiligo.

4. **What is the next best step?**

In this case, the most appropriate course of action for the patient would be to offer reassurance, given that a clinical evaluation is usually sufficient to diagnose vitiligo.

However, if the diagnosis remained uncertain, further assessment of the affected areas could be accomplished with a Wood's lamp examination. This procedure would provide a more detailed analysis of the extent of epidermal pigmentation loss, with greater contrast of the affected area in comparison to normal skin indicating a more significant loss. In patients with vitiligo, a Wood's lamp examination would reveal a fluorescent chalk-white to blue-white color over the depigmented lesions.[3]

5. **What are the most appropriate diagnostic modalities (i.e., labs, biopsies, scrapings, histological findings)?**

The diagnosis of vitiligo can usually be established clinically based on the characteristic appearance of depigmented patches on the skin.[5] However, diagnostic modalities may be necessary in certain instances either to confirm the diagnosis or to evaluate for the presence of associated autoimmune conditions. Appropriate diagnostic tests in such scenarios include a skin biopsy and blood tests to search for autoantibodies. Some recommended autoantibodies to screen for include serum antithyroglobulin, antithyroid peroxidase, and antinuclear antibodies.[5]

6. **What would you expect to find on histopathologic analysis?**

   On a histopathological level, the biopsy of an area of depigmented skin in a patient with vitiligo would reveal a complete absence of both melanocytes and melanin at the junction between the dermis and epidermis. Occasionally, lymphocytic infiltration can also be observed at the edges of the lesions.[4] Histology would otherwise be normal.

7. **Discuss the epidemiology of this disease**.

   a. **Discuss the incidence and prevalence:**

      The prevalence of vitiligo is roughly 1% within the United States and Europe but varies from 0.1% to 8% worldwide.[1]

   b. **Discuss the sociodemographics of individuals affected by this disease (i.e., age, gender, race, geographic location, other risk factors):**

      Vitiligo affects both sexes equally; however, due to the increased willingness of women to voice cosmetic concerns, females may be overrepresented in reported cases.[1] The disease affects half of all patients before the age of 20. Although late onset of vitiligo can occur in older patients, this is uncommon and may indicate the presence of autoimmune conditions such as diabetes mellitus, thyroid dysfunction, rheumatoid arthritis, and alopecia areata.[1] Additionally, approximately one-fifth of individuals with vitiligo have a family member with the same condition. In fact, the chance of first-degree relatives developing vitiligo are 7–10 times higher than those without a family history of the disease.[7]

8. **Discuss the pathogenesis of this disease**.

   Vitiligo is caused by the destruction of functional melanocytes in the epidermis. However, considering the observed diversity in the clinical presentations of vitiligo, it is highly probable that the underlying causes of the disease may differ among individuals and are multifaceted.[4] As a result, various theories have been proposed to explain the pathogenesis. Namely, the autoimmune theory proposes that particular melanocytes are targeted and destroyed by activated cytotoxic lymphocytes. Meanwhile, the self-destruct hypothesis postulates that toxic compounds are produced during melanin synthesis, which may play a role in triggering autoimmune destruction of melanocytes.[6] Additionally, the neurogenic hypothesis suggests that the developmental origin of melanocytes from neural crest cells plays a role in the pigmentation abnormalities seen in patients with vitiligo.[5]

9. **What is the clinical presentation of this disease (i.e., grade, stage, subtypes)?**

   The clinical presentation of vitiligo is variable and patient specific (Table 13.2).

Table 13.2   Classification of Vitiligo

TYPE	SUBTYPE	COMMENTS
Non-segmental vitiligo (NSV)	**Generalized**	Greater than 20% of body surface area is affected. Lesions are generally symmetrical.[8]
	Universal	80–90% of body surface area is affected. Most common form of vitiligo in adults.[8]
	Acrofacial	Depigmented macules present on face, hands, and feet.
	Mucosal	Multiple mucosal surfaces of the body (i.e., lips and genitalia) contain depigmented macules.
Segmental vitiligo (SV)	**Uni-, bi- or multi-segmental**	Depigmentation involves either ≥1 dermatome or ≥1 side that respects the body's midline.[8]
Mixed (SV and NSV)	—	Initially, SV present, then over time NSV occurs symmetrically on both halves of the body.[9]
Unclassified or indeterminate	**Focal**	Only one site on the body contains a depigmented lesion, which is present for 1–2 years. May evolve into SV or NSV over time, necessitating a change in classification.[9]

10. Discuss treatment options.

The objective of vitiligo treatment is two-fold: to halt disease progression and to promote the restoration of pigmentation.[3] This is accomplished through the usage of immunosuppressant medications, phototherapy, and surgery.[10] It is important that the treatment of vitiligo be personalized to each patient according to factors such as the patient's age and motivation for treatment as well as the extent, progression, and subtype of their disease.[3,7]

Overall, the treatment modality most frequently used for vitiligo is ultraviolet (UV) light therapy, as it stimulates repigmentation. Studies suggest that combining this therapy with another treatment modality can lead to better outcomes.[7] In patients with focal lesions, topical administration of agents such as a calcineurin inhibitor (TCI), corticosteroid (TCS), or a topical photochemotherapeutic agent such as 8-methoxypsoralen could cause pigment to return to the skin.[6] However, patients with generalized vitiligo benefit from treatment modalities that are systemic and used for longer periods. In these patients, oral psoralens may be used for a minimum of 1 year to achieve repigmentation of up to 85% of vitiligo lesions on the trunk, proximal extremities, head, and neck.[5,6] Unfortunately, the distal extremities do not respond well to psoralen combined UVA (PUVA) irradiation.

Recently, the U.S. Food and Drug Administration approved topical ruxolitinib, a JAK 1 and 2 inhibitor, for the treatment of non-segmental vitiligo in patients aged 12 or older.[11] The lotion lowers immune response by suppressing interferon (IFN)-γ signaling, promoting healthy skin cell development, and reintroducing pigment to affected areas, producing an even skin tone.[7,11,12] In clinical trials, the topical form was more efficacious than oral forms and had a better safety profile; however, systemic JAK inhibitors are still utilized off-label by some providers.[12] Adverse effects have been observed for the topical form, and further research is needed to determine its efficacy and safety.[11]

Additionally, surgical mini-grafting techniques can be utilized in cosmetically sensitive areas for patients who have stable disease, refractory hypopigmentation after 1 year of medical intervention, and no evidence of Koebner's phenomenon. The goal of these procedures is to relocate a healthy supply of melanocytes to affected areas so they can grow and move into areas where pigmentation is needed.[5,7]

An option reserved for adults with severe vitiligo who have failed other treatments and desire uniformity in their skin color is monobenzylether of hydroquinone (MEH) 20% cream. This cream causes the permanent depigmentation of normal skin as melanocytes are destroyed by the phenolic toxin in the product.[5]

11. Other important questions/details
Koebner's phenomenon
In some patients with vitiligo, isomorphic depigmented lesions tend to appear in areas of the body that have been subject to mechanical trauma. Notably, prior to traumatization, these cutaneous sites are known to be uninvolved with the disease.[9] This suggests that mechanical stress can induce vitiligo in a number of patients with the condition.

References

1. Alikhan A, Felsten LM, Daly M, Petronic-Rosic V. Vitiligo: A comprehensive overview part I. Introduction, epidemiology, quality of life, diagnosis, differential diagnosis, associations, histopathology, etiology, and work-up. *J Am Acad Dermatol*. 2011;65(3):473–491.
2. Stowman AM. Educational case: Vitiligo. *Acad Pathol*. 2019;6:2374289519888719.
3. Bolognia JL, Jorizzo JL, Schaffer JV. *Dermatology*. Vol 2, 3rd ed. Philadelphia: Elsevier Saunders; 2012.
4. Yaghoobi R, Omidian M, Bagherani N. Vitiligo: A review of the published work. *J Dermatol*. 2011;38(5):419–431.
5. Halder RM, Chappell JL. Vitiligo update. *Semin Cutan Med Surg*. 2009;28(2):86–92.
6. Wolff K, Johnson RA, Saavedra AP, Roh EK. *Fitzpatrick's Color Atlas and Synopsis of Clinical Dermatology*. New York: McGraw-Hill Education; 2017.
7. Bergqvist C, Ezzedine K. Vitiligo: A review. *Dermatology*. 2020;236(6):571–592.
8. Faria AR, Tarlé RG, Dellatorre G, Mira MT, Castro CC. Vitiligo—Part 2—Classification, histopathology and treatment. *An Bras Dermatol*. 2014;89(5):784–790.
9. Ezzedine K, Lim HW, Suzuki T, et al. Revised classification/nomenclature of vitiligo and related issues: The vitiligo global issues consensus conference. *Pigment Cell Melanoma Res*. 2012;25(3):E1–E13.
10. Kawakami T, Hashimoto T. Disease severity indexes and treatment evaluation criteria in vitiligo. *Dermatol Res Pract*. 2011;2011:750342.
11. Sheikh A, Rafique W, Owais R, Malik F, Ali E. FDA approves ruxolitinib (opzelura) for vitiligo therapy: A breakthrough in the field of dermatology. *Ann Med Surg (Lond)*. 2022;81:104499.
12. Qi F, Liu F, Gao L. Janus kinase inhibitors in the treatment of vitiligo: A review. *Front Immunol*. 2021;12:790125.

14

RED, SCALY SPOTS

DIVYA M. SHAN

A 17-year-old male presents to the clinic with multiple thick, well-demarcated, erythematous patches of skin with silvery scales (Figure 14.1). They cover his elbows and part of his scalp. The patient states that the lesions are itchy and notices bleeding with excessive scratching of the lesions. The lesions have caused him to feel very self-conscious. He has tried applying moisturizer in the affected areas and switching soaps with no major improvement. He notes that the lesions worsen around the time of stressful events such as final exams. The patient's family history reveals a grandfather who had recurrent episodes of similar lesions.

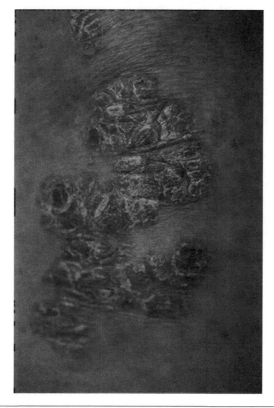

Figure 14.1 Patient presentation.

DOI: 10.1201/9781003437987-14

1. **How would you describe the lesions?**

   There are multiple well-defined, erythematous plaques covered in silvery-white scales on the elbows and scalp.

2. **What are the differential diagnoses?**

   There are numerous conditions to consider when establishing a diagnosis for a red, scaly rash (Table 14.1). Obtaining complete family, medical, and social histories, as well as performing a thorough physical examination, will help establish the diagnosis.

Table 14.1   Differential Diagnoses for Red, Scaly Rash

DIAGNOSIS	COMMENTS
Psoriasis	Symmetric distribution of well-demarcated, erythematous plaques covered in silvery scales that typically present on the extensor surfaces, scalp, and lower back. Often associated with pruritus.[1]
Atopic dermatitis	Presents as scaly, erythematous plaques and is classically associated with pruritus and personal or family history of atopic conditions such as allergic rhinitis or asthma.[2]
Lichen simplex chronicus	Manifests as lichenified, scaly plaques due to repeated scratching.[3]
Lichen planus	Violaceous, polygonal papules and plaques with fine white lines called Wickham striae. The lesions are pruritic and often involve mucous membranes, especially the mouth.[4]
Nummular dermatitis	Coin-shaped, eczematous, pruritic lesions that primarily occur on the extremities.[5]
Tinea infections	Annular, scaly, erythematous plaques with central clearing. Can occur on various locations such as the scalp, groin, foot, or other body surfaces. Diagnosis can be confirmed with potassium hydroxide (KOH) preparation.[6,7]
Drug eruption	A drug either initiates or aggravates skin lesions, which can vary in appearance, but can present with red, scaly, and raised patches or plaques.[8]
Pityriasis rubra pilaris	Follicular papules that coalesce to form red-orange, scaly plaques with islands of sparing, as well as keratoderma of the palms and soles.[9]
Pityriasis lichenoides chronica	Small, red-brown papules with central scale followed by hypo/hyperpigmentation.[10]
Subacute cutaneous lupus erythematosus	Annular, scaly, erythematous plaques in sun-exposed areas.[11] Associated with positive antinuclear antibodies (ANAs), anti-dsDNA, and anti-Smith antibodies.
Mycosis fungoides	Disease has an indolent course and presents as erythematous, scaly plaques. Classic findings include lymphadenopathy, leonine facies, and numerous atypical lymphocytes.[12]

3. **What is the most likely diagnosis?**

   The most likely diagnosis given the morphology of the lesions and patient history is psoriasis. The lesions may present anywhere on the body but are often found on the extensor surfaces of the elbows and knees, lower back, and scalp as seen in this patient. Tobacco use and family history of psoriasis are both factors that further support this diagnosis.[13]

4. **What is the next best step?**

   Careful examination of the skin lesions is the best method to diagnose psoriasis. The lesions are often symmetrically distributed and present as well-circumscribed, erythematous, scaly plaques. Nail findings, as well as the involvement of the skin in the umbilicus and/or gluteal cleft, are specific signs for the diagnosis of psoriasis.[1] Although psoriasis is typically a clinical diagnosis, a skin biopsy can be performed to confirm the diagnosis if still unclear.[14] If patients report additional symptoms such as morning stiffness or swollen/tender joints, consider bone scans, ultrasound, or referral to a rheumatologist.[15] Gathering a comprehensive history of medications may help in determining the cause and treatment for the lesions.

5. **What are the most appropriate diagnostic modalities (i.e., labs, biopsies, scrapings, histological findings)?**

   Psoriasis is a clinical diagnosis—the most critical step in diagnosing this disease is careful evaluation of the skin lesions. Severity can be described (often for insurance coverage purposes) by percent body surface area affected (more than 5–10% is generally regarded as severe). The Psoriasis Area and Severity Index (PASI) can be used to grade the severity of the lesions by assessing factors such as body surface area, erythema, induration, and scaling; this index is typically used in research settings rather than clinical practice.[1] In more atypical or uncertain presentations of psoriasis, a biopsy can be performed.

6. **What would you expect to find in the histopathologic analysis?**

   On histopathologic analysis of the plaques, you would expect to see epidermal hyperplasia with elongation of rete ridges and dermal papillae. Histopathology would also reveal parakeratosis with collections of neutrophils (Munro's microabscesses), thinning of the suprapapillary plates, dilated capillaries in the dermal papillae, and neutrophils within the spinous layer (spongiform pustules of Kogoj). These latter four features are most useful in diagnosing psoriasis with histopathology. Similar findings are seen in fungal infections; special stain for fungus can help exclude fungal infection.[16]

7. **Discuss the epidemiology of this disease.**

   a. **Discuss the incidence and prevalence:**

      Psoriasis affects individuals worldwide, and its prevalence varies among different populations, with higher frequency in countries that are farther away from the equator.[17] In the United States, the prevalence of psoriasis is approximately 2%, with 150,000 new cases of psoriasis diagnosed each year.[18]

   b. **Discuss the sociodemographics of individuals affected by this disease (i.e., age, gender, race, geographic location, other risk factors):**

      Although psoriasis affects individuals of all ages, it has a bimodal distribution with peaks in the age groups 15–20 years and 55–60 years. It is equally prevalent in both males and females.[19] The rates of psoriasis are highest in Norway and nearly absent in American Samoa and among Indians of South America.[18]

Important risk factors for psoriasis include smoking and family history.[13] The genetic component for psoriasis has been well-demonstrated with a three-fold increased risk of psoriasis in monozygotic twins compared to fraternal twins and familial recurrence.

8. Discuss the pathogenesis of this disease.

Although the pathogenesis of psoriasis is not completely understood, it is most likely an immune-mediated condition due to multiple factors such as genetics and environmental triggers (i.e., trauma, infections, stress). Genomic studies have identified over 80 susceptibility alleles associated with psoriasis.[20] Continuous inflammation leads to the proliferation and altered differentiation of keratinocytes.

Among the genes linked to psoriasis are several immune signaling genes including genes for both subunits of interleukin (IL)-23, the IL-23 receptor, and tyrosine kinase 2 (TYK2).

9. What is the clinical presentation of this disease (i.e., grade, stage, subtypes)?

There are many clinical manifestations of psoriasis, with plaque psoriasis being the most common (Table 14.2).[21]

Table 14.2 Clinical Types of Psoriasis

PSORIASIS TYPE	DESCRIPTION
Plaque psoriasis	Well-demarcated, erythematous, scaly plaques on the extensor surfaces of the extremities, trunk, and scalp.
Pustular psoriasis	Recurrent episodes of widespread rash and sterile, neutrophil-rich pustules that can be associated with general symptoms (e.g., fever).[22]
Guttate psoriasis	Acute onset of small, drop-like papules that typically occurs in children after streptococcal infections.
Nail psoriasis	Psoriasis in the nails manifests as pitting, onycholysis, and splinter hemorrhages.[23]
Erythrodermic psoriasis	A generalized form of psoriasis that affects over 80% of the body surface and presents as large, erythematous patches.
Psoriatic arthritis	Psoriasis associated with inflammatory arthritis and an absence of rheumatoid factor. It is associated with HLA-B27.[24]

Psoriasis has typically been categorized based on the percentage of involvement of the total body surface area. Mild psoriasis covers less than 3% of the body surface area, moderate psoriasis covers 3–10% of the body, and severe psoriasis covers more than 10% of the body.[25] Involvement of the face, genitals, and/or palms and soles is generally considered severe as well.

10. Discuss treatment options.

The treatment options for psoriasis vary based on the disease severity and can be organized as topical therapies, phototherapy, and systemic therapies

(Table 14.3).[26] In the context of treatment planning, psoriasis can be dichotomized into mild versus moderate-to-severe psoriasis. Mild psoriasis is often treated with topical therapy alone, while moderate-to-severe psoriasis may need phototherapy or systemic treatment. Selection of specific agents is dependent on numerous factors such as insurance coverage, adverse effects, comorbidities, and response to prior therapies.[27]

For mild psoriasis, the first-line agent is topical corticosteroids. Alternative therapies include vitamin D analogs and retinoids (e.g., tazarotene), which are more effective when combined with corticosteroids than alone.[28] Combination products such as calcipotriene-betamethasone and halobetasol-tazarotene are commercially available.[29] Localized phototherapy may be used in refractory cases of mild psoriasis. For moderate-to-severe psoriasis, treatment may involve phototherapy and systemic treatment. Ultraviolet B (UVB) is a first-line phototherapy for psoriasis, while psoralen plus ultraviolet A (PUVA) and pulsed dye laser (PDL) are second line.[30] Systemic agents such as methotrexate are the first-line systemic treatment for psoriasis, while newer biologic agents are used in refractory cases.[31]

It is important to schedule follow-up visits after the initial appointment to monitor the success of the treatment. Furthermore, early follow-up visits can improve patient adherence.[32]

Table 14.3   Therapies for Psoriasis

TREATMENT CATEGORY	EXAMPLES
Topical therapies	Corticosteroids
	Vitamin D analogs (calcipotriene, calcitriol)
	Calcineurin inhibitors
	Tar
	Tazarotene
	Tapinarof
	Roflumilast
	Anthralin
Phototherapy	Ultraviolet B (UVB)
	Psoralen plus ultraviolet A (PUVA)
	Pulsed dye laser (PDL)
	Excimer
Systemic therapies	Methotrexate
	Apremilast (phosphodiesterase-4 inhibitor)
	Cyclosporin
	Acitretin
	Deucravacitinib (TYK2 inhibitor)
	Biologic agents (tumor necrosis factor [TNF]-α inhibitors, interleukin [IL]-17 inhibitors, IL-23 inhibitors)

11. Other important questions/details:
    a. What outcomes can the patient expect and along what timeline?

Psoriasis is a chronic, recurrent inflammatory disease. Appropriate treatment can help control the disease process and avoid severe exacerbations. Some patients undergoing treatment may even achieve remission, defined as clear skin with no symptoms. However, patients who achieve remission are still at risk for recurrence of the disease. Given the unpredictable nature of psoriasis, it is difficult to predict how long remission will last.[33] Thus, patients should be provided with realistic expectations for managing their psoriasis. It will also be helpful to identify triggers of psoriasis in patients and avoid them.

With proper adherence to therapies, patients with mild psoriasis may see considerable improvement in 1 week and full benefits after several weeks. Patients with moderate-to-severe psoriasis usually see improvement in weeks.[33] With several types of treatments, including topical therapies, phototherapy, and systemic therapies, patients should be reassured that there are other options if they do not respond well to their initial treatment regimen. Patients should be routinely monitored for any adverse effects and promptly switched to a different treatment regimen if they experience any dermatological or systemic adverse effects.

Adherence to medication plays a critical role in the outcome of patients with chronic skin conditions.[34] Unfortunately, adherence rates to topical treatments can be abysmal.[35] Thus, taking measures to help improve adherence, such as scheduling an early follow-up, is important in achieving the best treatment outcomes.[32]

References

1. Kimmel GW, Lebwohl M. Psoriasis: Overview and diagnosis. In: Bhutani T, Liao W, Nakamura M, eds. *Evidence-Based Psoriasis*. Updates in Clinical Dermatology. Springer International Publishing; 2018:1–16.
2. Ahn C, Huang W. Clinical presentation of atopic dermatitis. In: Fortson EA, Feldman SR, Strowd LC, eds. *Management of Atopic Dermatitis*. Vol 1027. Advances in Experimental Medicine and Biology. Springer International Publishing; 2017:39–46.
3. Voicu C, Tebeica T, Zanardelli M, et al. Lichen simplex chronicus as an essential part of the dermatologic masquerade. *Open Access Maced J Med Sci*. 2017;5(4):556–557.
4. Wagner G, Rose C, Sachse MM. Clinical variants of lichen planus: Lichen planus. *JDDG J Dtsch Dermatol Ges*. 2013;11(4):309–319.
5. Leung AKC, Lam JM, Leong KF, Leung AAM, Wong AHC, Hon KL. Nummular eczema: An updated review. *Recent Pat Inflamm Allergy Drug Discov*. 2021;14(2):146–155.
6. Ely JW, Rosenfeld S, Seabury Stone M. Diagnosis and management of tinea infections. *Am Fam Physician*. 2014;90(10):702–710.
7. Leung AK, Lam JM, Leong KF, Hon KL. Tinea corporis: An updated review. *Drugs Context*. 2020;9:1–12.

8. Kim GK, Del Rosso JQ. Drug-provoked psoriasis: Is it drug induced or drug aggravated? Understanding pathophysiology and clinical relevance. *J Clin Aesthetic Dermatol.* 2010;3(1):32–38.

9. Wang D, Chong VCL, Chong WS, Oon HH. A review on pityriasis rubra pilaris. *Am J Clin Dermatol.* 2018;19(3):377–390.

10. Khachemoune A, Blyumin ML. Pityriasis lichenoides: Pathophysiology, classification, and treatment. *Am J Clin Dermatol.* 2007;8(1):29–36.

11. Eastham AB, Vleugels RA. Cutaneous lupus erythematosus. *JAMA Dermatol.* 2014;150(3):344.

12. Doukaki S, Aricò M, Bongiorno MR. A rare presentation of mycosis fungoides mimicking psoriasis vulgaris. *Case Rep Dermatol.* 2009;1(1):60–65.

13. Naldi L, Parazzini F, Brevi A, et al. Family history, smoking habits, alcohol consumption and risk of psoriasis. *Br J Dermatol.* 1992;127(3):212–217.

14. Alenius GM, Stenberg B, Stenlund H, Lundblad M, Dahlqvist SR. Inflammatory joint manifestations are prevalent in psoriasis: prevalence study of joint and axial involvement in psoriatic patients, and evaluation of a psoriatic and arthritic questionnaire. *J Rheumatol.* 2002;29(12):2577–2582.

15. Ory PA, Gladman DD, Mease PJ. Psoriatic arthritis and imaging. *Ann Rheum Dis.* 2005;64(Suppl 2):ii55–ii57.

16. Murphy M, Kerr P, Grant-Kels JM. The histopathologic spectrum of psoriasis. *Clin Dermatol.* 2007;25(6):524–528.

17. Parisi R, Symmons DPM, Griffiths CEM, Ashcroft DM. Global epidemiology of psoriasis: A systematic review of incidence and prevalence. *J Invest Dermatol.* 2013;133(2):377–385.

18. Gudjonsson JE, Elder JT. Psoriasis: Epidemiology. *Clin Dermatol.* 2007;25(6):535–546.

19. Eder L, Widdifield J, Rosen CF, et al. Trends in the prevalence and incidence of psoriasis and psoriatic arthritis in Ontario, Canada: A population-based study. *Arthritis Care Res.* 2019;71(8):1084–1091.

20. Ran D, Cai M, Zhang X. Genetics of psoriasis: A basis for precision medicine. *Precis Clin Med.* 2019;2(2):120–130.

21. Sarac G, Koca TT, Baglan T. A brief summary of clinical types of psoriasis. *North Clin Istanb.* 2016;3(1):79–82.

22. Marrakchi S, Puig L. Pathophysiology of generalized pustular psoriasis. *Am J Clin Dermatol.* 2022;23(S1):13–19.

23. Edwards F, De Berker D. Nail psoriasis: Clinical presentation and best practice recommendations. *Drugs.* 2009;69(17):2351–2361.

24. Gladman DD. Psoriatic arthritis. *Dermatol Ther.* 2009;22(1):40–55.

25. Lewis-Beck C, Abouzaid S, Xie L, Baser O, Kim E. Analysis of the relationship between psoriasis symptom severity and quality of life, work productivity, and activity impairment among patients with moderate-to-severe psoriasis using structural equation modeling. *Patient Prefer Adherence.* 2013;7:199–205.

26. Elmets CA, Korman NJ, Prater EF, et al. Joint AAD-NPF guidelines of care for the management and treatment of psoriasis with topical therapy and alternative medicine modalities for psoriasis severity measures. *J Am Acad Dermatol.* 2021;84(2):432–470.

27. Kim WB, Jerome D, Yeung J. Diagnosis and management of psoriasis. *Can Fam Physician Med Fam Can.* 2017;63(4):278–285.

28. Hendriks AGM, Keijsers RRMC, De Jong EMGJ, Seyger MMB, Van De Kerkhof PCM. Efficacy and safety of combinations of first-line topical treatments in chronic plaque psoriasis: A systematic literature review: Systematic review on combinations of first-line topicals. *J Eur Acad Dermatol Venereol.* 2013;27(8):931–951.

29. Wu JJ, Hansen JB, Patel DS, Nyholm N, Veverka KA, Swensen AR. Effectiveness comparison and incremental cost-per-responder analysis of calcipotriene 0.005%/betamethasone dipropionate 0.064% foam vs. halobetasol 0.01%/tazarotene 0.045% lotion for plaque psoriasis: A matching-adjusted indirect comparative analysis. *J Med Econ.* 2020;23(6):641–649.
30. Zhang P, Wu MX. A clinical review of phototherapy for psoriasis. *Lasers Med Sci.* 2018;33(1):173–180.
31. Balak DMW. First-line systemic treatment of psoriasis: Staying conventional or going biologic? *Br J Dermatol.* 2017;177(4):897–898.
32. Davis SA, Lin HC, Yu CH, Balkrishnan R, Feldman SR. Underuse of early follow-up visits: A missed opportunity to improve patients' adherence. *J Drugs Dermatol JDD.* 2014;13(7):833–836.
33. Lebwohl M. A clinician's paradigm in the treatment of psoriasis. *J Am Acad Dermatol.* 2005;53(1):S59–S69.
34. Carroll CL, Feldman SR, Camacho FT, Balkrishnan R. Better medication adherence results in greater improvement in severity of psoriasis. *Br J Dermatol.* 2004;151(4):895–897.
35. Zschocke I, Mrowietz U, Karakasili E, Reich K. Non-adherence and measures to improve adherence in the topical treatment of psoriasis. *J Eur Acad Dermatol Venereol.* 2014;28:4–9.

15

PAINFUL, ERYTHEMATOUS NODULES

ADITI CHOKSHI

A 32-year-old Caucasian female with a history of diabetes presents to the clinic with persistent painful "boils" in the left axilla that started 2 weeks previously (Figure 15.1). She reports a foul odor and states that the lesions intermittently drain "white fluid." The patient has a history of similar lesions in both axillae and medial thighs since the age of 20. She states she has not sought medical care because the lesions typically resolve spontaneously. Her only medication is metformin. The patient currently smokes one pack of cigarettes and drinks one to two beers a night. She has a 10-pack-year history of cigarette smoking and has a body mass index (BMI) of 28 kg/m². Examination reveals malodorous, painful, erythematous nodules with thick bands of scar tissue.

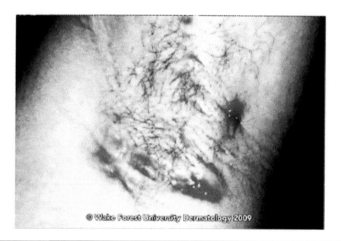

Figure 15.1 Patient presentation.

1. How would you describe the lesions?

The lesions are dispersed over the left axilla with several painful, erythematous nodules with purulent drainage measuring approximately 1–2 cm in diameter. Sinus tract formation, dermal contractures, and scarring are evident in the center of the lesions.

   DOI: 10.1201/9781003437987-15

2. What are the differential diagnoses (Table 15.1)?

Table 15.1 Differential Diagnoses for Painful, Erythematous Nodules

DIAGNOSIS	COMMENTS
Inflamed epidermal inclusion cyst	Epidermal cysts can rupture and become inflamed and begin to have purulent drainage. Epidermal cysts are typically solitary lesions that present with a central punctum and can be located anywhere on the body, including the face, neck, trunk, genitalia, and buccal mucosa.[1]
Nodulocystic acne	Nodulocystic acne presents as inflamed nodules, cysts, and comedones distributed along the face, upper back, and chest.[1] The lesions are confined to the superficial compartment and convex skin surfaces.[2]
Furuncles/ carbuncles	Furuncles present as inflamed, painful, fluctuant abscesses that can coalesce to form a larger nodule known as a carbuncle. Furuncles and carbuncles are transient and respond well with antibiotic therapy.[3] Furuncles and carbuncles are due to an infectious etiology, most commonly *Staphylococcus aureus*.[3]
Crohn's disease	Cutaneous manifestations of Crohn's disease include anal canal fissures that can progress to fistula and sinus tract formation. Crohn's disease occurs in young adulthood and is linked to tobacco smoking and an abnormal inflammatory response. Crohn's disease is characterized by gastrointestinal symptoms of persistent diarrhea, abdominal bloating, and cramps. Lesions are limited to the perianal or anal area.[1]
Infected Bartholin's gland	Bartholin cysts are located on the posterior introitus at the base of the labia majora. Bartholin cysts are asymptomatic in the majority of women, but may present with painful intercourse, genital pain, or pain while walking or sitting. A minority of patients may develop a fever if an abscess develops. Treatment of Bartholin cysts with fistulization and placement of a Word catheter results in resolution and low recurrence rates.[4]
Hidradenitis suppurativa	HS is a chronic, inflammatory disorder affecting the axillae, groin, buttocks, and inframammary creases.[1] The lesions in HS involve the deep part of the hair follicle.[2] The exact pathogenesis of HS is unclear; however, a widely accepted theory proposes that the development of lesions is due to an inflammatory etiology involving follicular plugging and dilation of the pilosebaceous unit leading to influx of inflammatory cells and abscess formation.[5] HS is characterized by a recurrent course with development of long-term complications such as scarring, sinus tracts, and edema from obstruction of lymphatics by scar tissue despite treatment with antibiotics.[6]

HS: Hidradenitis suppurativa

3. What is the most likely diagnosis?

The most likely diagnosis in this patient is hidradenitis suppurativa (HS).

4. What is the next best step?

The next best step in the management of these lesions is to evaluate the disease severity via the Hurley classification (Table 15.2) to decide on the appropriate treatment plan. Mild, stage 1 lesions can be managed with topical antibiotics such as clindamycin and counseling on lifestyle modifications, including abstinence from smoking, weight loss, and avoidance of

Table 15.2 Hurley Classification System[7]

HURLEY STAGE	CHARACTERISTICS
I	• Single or multiple abscesses • No evidence of sinus tracts, fistulas, or scarring
II	• Single or multiple abscesses with evidence of sinus tracts and scarring in one or more areas of the body
III	• Multiple interconnected sinus tracts, fissures, and abscesses with diffuse involvement of skin

tight clothing. However, severe stage 3 lesions, as seen in our patient, may benefit from treatment with biologics, immunosuppressants, or retinoids. If no improvement is seen with medications, operative interventions such as surgical excisions, incision and drainage, or carbon dioxide laser excisions may be considered.[5,6]

5. **What are the most appropriate diagnostic modalities (i.e., labs, biopsies, scrapings, histological findings)?**

HS is a clinical diagnosis and often misdiagnosed. The consensus diagnostic criteria require patients to have evidence of all three criteria:

1) Typical lesions and morphology such as painful nodules, sinus tract formation, abscesses, or scarring
2) Typical distribution of lesions in axillae, inguinal, perianal, and inframammary folds
3) History of recurrence and chronic lesions, defined as more than two lesions in 6 months[7]

If the diagnosis is unclear or the lesions are unresponsive to treatment, the diagnosis may be confirmed by other diagnostic modalities (Table 15.3).

Table 15.3   Diagnostic Modalities for Hidradenitis Suppurativa

DIAGNOSTIC MODALITIES	DETAILS
Color Doppler ultrasound	Doppler ultrasound can allow for earlier recognition of changes such as dermal thickening, pseudocysts, expansion of hair follicles, and fluid collections that would not be visualized on clinical examination.[7] Ultrasound can also be utilized to detect deep, unruptured HS lesions and sinus tracts that are not palpable on physical exam. Some clinicians believe that diagnosis via ultrasound is more accurate than with Hurley staging due to earlier detection of lesions and the increased accuracy in categorization of patients based on disease severity.[8]
Skin biopsy	Histologic analysis of HS lesions is not diagnostic but can aid in ruling out other diseases. Skin biopsies of lesions are not recommended unless the lesions are atypical or not responding to multiple treatment modalities. Histologic findings of HS include follicular hyperkeratosis and plugging, lymphocytic inflammatory infiltrate, abscess formation, and sinus tracts with stratified squamous epithelium and fibrosis.[9] Histology may also be useful in identifying the onset of sinus tract formation with visualization of psoriasiform hyperplasia and low-grade leukocytic infiltrate in the perilesional dermis.[8]
Laboratory testing	In patients who develop abnormal HS lesions with atypical morphology or distribution, a complete blood count (CBC), qualitative immunoglobulin testing (IgA, IgM, IgG, and IgE levels), complement levels, and HIV testing may be performed to identify immunocompromised patients.[6]

6. **What would you expect to find in the histopathologic analysis?**

HS is typically diagnosed via thorough history and physical examination. However, a skin biopsy can be performed for atypical HS presentations or if lesions are unresponsive to treatment. Histologic findings of HS include follicular hyperkeratosis and plugging, lymphocytic inflammatory infiltrate, abscess formation, and sinus tracts with stratified squamous epithelium and fibrosis.[9]

7. **Discuss the epidemiology of this disease**
   a. **Discuss the incidence and prevalence:**
   The estimated prevalence rate for HS is 0.1% of the general population, with a predominance of females 18–40 years old.[1] Disease severity typically peaks in ages 30–40, with increased rates of resolution after menopause.[7]
   b. **Discuss the sociodemographics of individuals affected by this disease (i.e., age, gender, race, geographic location, other risk factors):**
   Obesity and cigarette smoking are two risk factors highly correlated with development of HS. Cigarette smoking may contribute to HS by promotion of epidermal hyperplasia and increasing the inflammatory response via mast cell degranulation and increased leukocyte chemotaxis.[6] Obesity results in a chronic low-grade inflammatory response, along with increased friction and stress in intertriginous areas. This increases follicular hyperkeratinization and occlusion of follicular ducts. Several studies have supported the finding of increased disease severity associated with increasing body mass index (BMI).[10] Genetic factors are strongly associated with the development of HS, with 33% of patients having a positive family history. Mutations in the gamma-secretase genes are hypothesized to promote atypical epidermal proliferation and differentiation.[7]

8. **Discuss the pathogenesis of this disease**.
   Although the exact pathogenesis of HS has not been established, there are several well-supported theories on the etiology of its development. Previously, HS development was believed to be due to an infectious etiology involving the apocrine sweat glands. However, immune dysregulation of the skin results in perifollicular inflammation, and blockage of hair follicles may contribute to HS lesion development.[7] Increasing occlusion of the hair follicular ducts results in subsequent rupture and leakage of keratin and bacteria into the surrounding dermal tissue. This stimulates an abundance of neutrophils and leukocytes to migrate to the tissue and the development of painful, erythematous nodules.[11] Chronic inflammation leads to fistula and sinus tract formation and provides an optimal environment for biofilm formation. Bacterial biofilms are difficult to eliminate and can lead to secondary infections, disease exacerbations, abscesses with purulent drainage, and diffuse involvement of the skin.[7]

9. **What is the clinical presentation of this disease (i.e., grade, stage, subtypes)?**
   HS presents as painful, erythematous nodules that, if left untreated, can progress to deep abscesses with purulent and malodorous drainage. HS is a chronic, relapsing disease characterized by recurrent flares and formation of dermal contractures and scarring.[7] The distribution of lesions is utilized to further classify the disease into three subtypes: axillary-mammary, follicular, and gluteal. However, there is no difference in treatment based on the subtype.[8]

10. **Discuss treatment options**.
    Treatment of HS is based on the stage of severity established by the Hurley classification system (Table 15.4). All patients should be informed of the benefits

of lifestyle modifications including smoking cessation, weight loss, hygiene, and avoidance of tight-fitting clothing.[5]

Stage 1 HS can be treated with topical clindamycin, antiseptics such as benzoyl peroxide, and intralesional corticosteroids. Incision and drainage, deroofing, or laser excision may be considered for persistent nodules.

Stage 2 HS was previously treated with doxycycline, though in recent studies there was no improvement in efficacy with doxycycline compared to topical clindamycin in stage 2 HS patients. Patients with stage 2 have achieved near-remission or significant resolution with combination treatment of clindamycin and rifampicin or triple therapy with rifampicin, moxifloxacin, and metronidazole. Immune modulators such as prednisolone and dapsone may also be considered but have mixed efficacy.[11] Deroofing and laser excision are surgical interventions that may be utilized if necessary.

Stage 3 HS is treated with biologics—although adalimumab and secukinumab are the only Food and Drug Administration (FDA)–approved biologics for HS, bimekizumab may be utilized as off-label treatment.[10,12] Surgical excision can be considered for severe cases with fistulas, sinus tracts, or extensive scarring.[10]

Although the mechanism in which hormones influence disease progression is not well understood, patients taking combination oral contraceptives (OCPs), spironolactone, and finasteride had improved outcomes, with 50% of patients having significant improvement or complete resolution of lesions. Patients with concurrent polycystic ovarian syndrome (PCOS) have benefitted the most from treatment with OCPs.[1]

Table 15.4   Treatment Options for Hidradenitis Suppurativa

HURLEY STAGE	TREATMENT	DOSING	MECHANISM OF ACTION
I	Topical clindamycin	• 0.1% applied twice daily for 6–8 weeks[6]	Binds to the 50s subunit of the bacterial ribosome, which inhibits peptide bond formation and protein synthesis
II	Doxycycline	• 100 mg twice daily[6]	Binds to the 30s ribosomal subunit, which inhibits bacterial protein synthesis
	Oral clindamycin	• 300 mg twice daily for 10 days[6]	Binds to the 50s subunit of the bacterial ribosome, which inhibits peptide bond formation and protein synthesis
	Rifampicin	• 600 mg twice daily (with clindamycin) for 10 days[6] • 10 mg/kg once daily (with moxifloxacin and metronidazole) for 6 weeks[11]	Inhibits bacterial DNA-dependent RNA polymerase and blocks elongation of RNA
	Moxifloxacin	• 400 mg once daily (with rifampicin and metronidazole) for 6 weeks[11]	Inhibits DNA gyrase enzyme and inhibits separation of bacterial DNA and cell replication
	Metronidazole	• 500 mg three times daily (with rifampicin and metronidazole) for 6 weeks[11]	Inhibits nucleic acid synthesis via the formation of free radicals and disruption of DNA in microbial cells

(Continued)

Table 15.4 (*Continued*)   Treatment Options for Hidradenitis Suppurativa

HURLEY STAGE	TREATMENT	DOSING	MECHANISM OF ACTION
	Prednisolone	• 10 mg once daily for 4–6 weeks[6]	Decreases inflammatory response via decreasing vasodilation and permeability of capillaries and decreasing leukocyte migration to inflammatory sites
	Dapsone	• 50–200 mg once daily for 3 weeks[6]	Inhibits bacterial synthesis of dihydrofolic acid via competition with para-amino-benzoate for the active site of dihydropteroate synthetase
III	Adalimumab	• 80 mg once weekly for the first 2 weeks followed by 40 mg once weekly for 24 weeks[1,6]	Recombinant human IgG1 monoclonal antibody that blocks interaction between TNF-α and its receptors
	Secukinumab	• 300 mg every 4 weeks, or every 2 weeks if inadequate response[12]	Inhibits IL-17A

mg: milligrams; **TNF:** tumor necrosis factor; **IL:** interleukin

11. **Other important questions/details:**

Complications

Untreated HS can result in secondary infections with abscess formation. Rarely, infections can progress to sepsis or erysipelas. Prolonged tissue inflammation can also result in development of anemia of chronic disease, hypoalbuminemia, or amyloidosis. Additionally, the psychological burden from chronic pain, malodorous discharge, and scarring in genital regions contributes to depression, sexual dysfunction, work disability, and lowered quality of life among patients.[7] However, complications of HS can be prevented with early diagnosis and prompt initiation of appropriate treatment.

Special populations

Pediatric HS is less common than adult HS but has similar long-term sequelae such as increased risk of metabolic syndrome, PCOS, and psychiatric disorders. Treatment of pediatric HS is the same as that for adult HS, but antibiotic treatment is limited to 6 months, and tetracyclines are contraindicated in children ages 9 or younger. In pregnant patients with HS, topical clindamycin or benzoyl peroxide may be used for mild disease. In severe disease, intravenous ertapenem or tumor necrosis factor (TNF)-α inhibitors such adalimumab or infliximab can be used in the first and second trimesters. Breastfeeding mothers are safe to continue treatment with clindamycin, rifampin, cephalexin, or amoxicillin.[1]

Chronic hidradenitis suppurativa

Severe, chronic HS can result in development of strictures, fistulas, and contractures with progression to limited limb mobility.[5,9] Chronic sustained inflammation can also lead to the development of lymphedema and squamous cell carcinoma, or vulvar squamous cell carcinoma if lesions involve the genitalia.[5,7]

References

1. Sayed CJ, Hsiao JL, Okun MM. Clinical epidemiology and management of hidradenitis suppurativa. *Obstet Gynecol.* 2021;137(4):731–746.
2. Fimmel S, Zouboulis CC. Comorbidities of hidradenitis suppurativa (acne inversa). *Dermatoendocrinol.* 2010;2(1):9–16.
3. Ibler KS, Kromann CB. Recurrent furunculosis—Challenges and management: A review. *Clin Cosmet Investig Dermatol.* 2014;7:59–64.
4. Omole F, Kelsey RC, Phillips K, Cunningham K. Bartholin duct cyst and gland abscess: Office management. *Am Fam Physician.* 2019;99(12):760–766.
5. Collier EK, Parvataneni RK, Lowes MA, et al. Diagnosis and management of hidradenitis suppurativa in women. *Am J Obstet Gynecol.* January, 2021;224(1):54–61.
6. Anduquia-Garay F, Rodríguez-Gutiérrez MM, Poveda-Castillo IT, et al. Hidradenitis suppurativa: Basic considerations for its approach: A narrative review. *Ann Med Surg (Lond).* August, 2021;68:102679.
7. Vinkel C, Thomsen SF. Hidradenitis suppurativa: Causes, features, and current treatments. *J Clin Aesthet Dermatol.* October, 2018;11(10):17–23.
8. Elkin K, Daveluy S, Avanaki K. Hidradenitis suppurativa: Current understanding, diagnostic and surgical challenges, and developments in ultrasound application. *Skin Res Technol.* 2019;26(1):11–19.
9. Micheletti, MDRG. Natural history, presentation, and diagnosis of hidradenitis suppurativa. *Semin Cutan Med Surg.* 2014;33(3S).
10. Scala E, Cacciapuoti S, Garzorz-Stark N, et al. Hidradenitis suppurativa: Where we are and where we are going. *Cells.* 2021;10(8).
11. Napolitano M, Megna M, Timoshchuk EA, et al. Hidradenitis suppurativa: From pathogenesis to diagnosis and treatment. *Clin Cosmet Investig Dermatol.* 2017;10:105–115.
12. Novartis. FDA approves Novartis Cosentyx® as the first new biologic treatment option for hidradenitis suppurativa patients in nearly a decade. *Novartis;* 2023. Accessed November 24, 2023. Available at: www.novartis.com/news/media-releases/fda-approves-novartis-cosentyx-first-new-biologic-treatment-option-hidradenitis-suppurativa-patients-nearly-decade.

Index

Note: Page numbers in *italics* indicate figures and those in **bold** indicate tables.

T - #0291 - 160425 - C136 - 254/178/7 - PB - 9781032571362 - Gloss Lamination